What Mental Illness Really Is...

(and what it isn't)

LUCY FOULKES

VINTAGE

1 3 5 7 9 10 8 6 4 2

Vintage is part of the Penguin Random House group of companies
whose addresses can be found at global.penguinrandomhouse.com

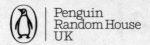

Penguin
Random House
UK

First published in Vintage in 2022
First published in hardback with the title *Losing Our Minds*
by The Bodley Head in 2021

penguin.co.uk/vintage

A CIP catalogue record for this book is available from the British Library

ISBN 9781529113372

Printed and bound in Great Britain by Clays Ltd, Elcograf S.p.A.

The authorised representative in the EEA is Penguin Random House Ireland,
Morrison Chambers, 32 Nassau Street, Dublin D02 YH68

Penguin Random House is committed to a sustainable future
for our business, our readers and our planet. This book is made
from Forest Stewardship Council® certified paper.

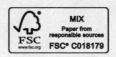

MIX
Paper from
responsible sources
FSC
www.fsc.org
FSC® C018179

Contents

A note on terminology

There is no uncontroversial language when talking about mental illness – and that includes the phrase 'mental illness'.

Nathan Filer

When it comes to matters of human distress, some people argue that the labels of 'illness' or 'disorder' are unhelpful, and I am entirely sympathetic to this view. The concern is that these terms are stigmatising and medicalising, implying entirely internal causes or personal fault when – as we will see – so many of these 'symptoms' are an understandable response to suffering and hardship brought on by stressful lives. But alongside this, I also believe that some psychological experiences are so distressing and disabling that the labels of illness and disorder can be useful and necessary. I therefore use these terms, cautiously, throughout this book. But I recognise that this language, like all language on this topic, is imperfect – and I talk about that quite a bit too.

INTRODUCTION

Collateral damage

Let me paint a picture of an idyllic life. It's my life, in fact, when I was twenty, in the summer after my second year at university. I was studying psychology, which I found fascinating. I had just started going out with my boyfriend, another student, and I was falling in love. I had a great summer job as a swimming teacher; I was close to my parents and my brother; I had a lovely bunch of friends both at university and at home. From the outside, my life that summer was incredibly easy, hopeful. But on the inside I was unravelling.

I was in Turkey when everything came undone, on the first night of a week-long holiday with my three best friends. The problem had been brewing for a while – I had been feeling low for months – but on that holiday a switch flicked in my head, and I suddenly became much, much worse. Walking back to our apartment after a day at the beach, seemingly out of nowhere, I began to feel like I couldn't breathe. My thoughts became dark and opaque. We found a doctor, and he said to me – in broken English, perplexed – 'Why you crying? You're on holiday.' He injected me with Valium, my friend beside me holding my hand. I flew home the following day, hoping vaguely that when I got home somehow everything would be okay. I was wrong. That summer was the start of months, of years, of my experience of mental illness.

When I walked into my kitchen after the flight, I had a strong sense that the room was unfamiliar. I knew objectively I was in my own house, but at the same time, it felt like I'd never been there before. (I later learnt this is called *derealisation*, or *jamais vu* – never seen – a sinister sister to the more common déjà vu.) It cloaked me like a cloud, a creeping, awful feeling, and I realised something serious was happening to me.

My dad took me to an out-of-hours clinic in a local hospital where I was prescribed more Valium, and then to a GP the following day, who gave me antidepressants. After the longest, darkest month of my life, I went back to university for my final year. I wasn't ready to go back, but I was too scared of the alternative: a year at home without distraction. At university I was a ghost in my own life: scared to be on my own; not sleeping; crying on campus and on trains.

It took about four months before I felt a glimmer of something that wasn't depression or anxiety, and about three years until I believed that those feelings wouldn't dominate my life. Over the years, I've seen many therapists and I also took medication on and off for about five years. I am much, much better now, and have periods where this all feels like a distant memory. But as anyone with similar experience will know: it lives with you.

But this book is not about me. There are plenty of excellent memoirs out there depicting what mental illness feels like, many of them by people who have suffered far more than I have. Instead, this book is about what's been happening around me: in the research world and in society at large. After I finished my degree – I did get there in the end – I decided to stay in academia, and I now have a PhD in psychology. I now work as an academic psychologist, researching mental illness, working with some of the most innovative mental health researchers in the world. This book is partly about this academic knowledge: mental illness is a fascinating, intricate, messy area of science, and there are so many stories about this research that need to be told. But something else has happened since I was first unwell, something in society, and the book is about that, too.

When it happened to me in 2008, no one talked about mental illness. The doctors and psychologists I saw told me it was very common, that they saw lots of patients with depression and anxiety, especially young people like me. When I looked around me, though, at society, at my peers, I saw nothing. There were some books, a few websites, but no *presence*, no public conversation. Professionals telling me that I wasn't alone was irrelevant, because everywhere I turned, in every practical respect, it felt like I was. However, this public silence was about to change. I didn't know it then, but my experience happened around the time of a significant cultural shift.

Campaign to destigmatise mental illness

It started in 2007, with a charity called Time to Change, whose goal was to end mental health discrimination and stigma. Their mission began quietly, but in 2011, they launched a national campaign, with four weeks of television adverts and the following tagline: 'It's time to talk. It's Time to Change.' Celebrities like Stephen Fry and Ruby Wax were involved, discussing their own mental illnesses. The campaign's flagship statistic – that one in four adults will experience a mental illness in any given year – started appearing widely. I clearly remember reading a Time to Change leaflet around then. I was working as a research assistant after my degree, and I used to go to secondary schools and ask teenage participants to complete a series of cognitive tasks on laptops. While waiting for one of them to finish, in an upstairs room of a maze-like old school, I started reading some of the health information on a noticeboard. One of the leaflets, bubblegum pink, was about the Time to Change campaign. I remember being struck by the one-in-four statistic, and the celebrity stories: realising there really were other people out there like me.

This campaign was a cultural turning point. From there, the momentum started to grow, a rumble in the background at first, gradually growing louder. More celebrities started admitting that they too had mental health problems – Davina McCall, Emma Stone, Lady Gaga. Famous and non-famous people alike starting writing memoirs; discussions of mental illness in the media exploded. People were getting trained in mental health awareness at work, children were learning about it in schools. Even the royal family got involved, with princes William and Harry encouraging us to open up when we're struggling. Now, we have Mental Health Awareness Week in May and World Mental Health Day in October. If that campaign was to get people talking about mental illness, then it worked: people are talking about it all right.

But there's a problem, and it's why I'm writing this book. The public understanding of mental illness is still limited. There's still a great deal of uncertainty about what disorders really involve, what causes them, and what the treatments are. We have become familiar with statistics about how common the problem is and hashtags encouraging us to open up to our friends. But this isn't enough. For starters, this message to speak about our mental illness is only useful if there is help at the other end: if the person *listening* actually understands what the problem is. And we're not there yet – very few people know how to respond to someone who is unwell. For all this drive to start talking, very few know how to listen; very few really know what it is they're supposed to say.

This is vital, because when a person has a mental illness, they need more than just professional help. In fact, psychological services are so underfunded and overstretched that a person will need a lot of informal support while waiting for professional help – if they are able to access it at all. They need support from many areas of their life: their place of work or study, their partner, their family, their friends. It's great that the essential first step has been taken, that the conversation has begun, but the public discourse around mental health now needs to go deeper, to recognise more fully what mental illness is. This will enable those suffering to not only understand themselves, but to be understood and supported by the people around them.

As an example, let's think about obsessive–compulsive disorder (OCD). The term OCD is very much in the public arena, often used casually, even flippantly, as a synonym for being organised or neat and tidy. In November 2016, for example, the *Telegraph* published an article entitled 'I have Obsessive–Christmas Disorder, and it's the greatest gift of all', which includes the twelve rules of this 'seasonal OCD'.[1] The first point is 'Make lists in a nice notebook'. In reality, OCD is a devastating mental illness, and it's worth taking a moment to explain exactly what it involves.

OCD has two components: intrusive repetitive thoughts (*obsessions*), and ritualistic behaviours or thoughts (*compulsions*) carried out to try and manage the distress caused by the obsessions. Imagine, for a moment, the most devastating or horrific thought possible. It might be about your loved ones dying, or about you hurting someone else. Or it might be deeply immoral, like something incestuous or paedophilic, or maybe something disgustingly unsanitary. These are all common intrusive thoughts among those with OCD, but there are others, and specific thoughts vary from person to person. In fact, having the occasional thought like this is pretty common: in a 2014 study of participants across the world, 94% reported at least one 'intrusive thought' in the past three months.[2] But now imagine – and this bit is critical – that instead of the horrific thought being fleeting, it's stuck on repeat in your head. It's as vivid as it would be if it was happening in front of you, and it won't go away. People with OCD in no way want these events to occur in real life, quite the opposite, but they are unable to stop imagining them. One mother with OCD has described experiencing endless violent intrusive thoughts about her baby. 'It's a horror movie that's going on in your head,' she said. 'This was a horror movie about my own son.'[3]

That's where the compulsions come in. These are actions carried out to temporarily relieve the anxiety caused by the intrusive thoughts. A sufferer who has intrusive thoughts about sanitation, for example, might repeatedly wash their hands. Note the word 'repeatedly': I knew someone with OCD who scrubbed their hands until they bled *and they still couldn't stop doing it.* Other people might carry out a system of checking and/or touching parts of their surroundings because their OCD has made them think this will prevent, for example, their family being harmed. Many compulsions are carried out privately, or performed only mentally, like counting or praying, but others are so conspicuous and attention-grabbing that the person cannot leave their home.

I talk more about OCD later in this book, but I use it here to illustrate a point: this disorder is awful, and not especially rare (the prevalence rate in the UK is around 1%[4]), but unless you're unlucky enough to have personally experienced it, the above description will likely come as new information. This is the problem: for all the awareness-raising – the fanfare and bunting and hashtags – there's still a lack of understanding of what disorders actually are, let alone why people get them or how we're supposed to help. We know mental illness exists, we know it's widespread, but few people really know what any of this *means*.

The absence of knowledge about mental health creates a vacuum that is filled by inaccuracies and half-truths. The casual misuse of the term OCD, for example, leads to a widespread and entrenched misunderstanding of what the disorder is. And it's not just OCD: it's bulimia, depression, bipolar disorder … these terms have been let loose into society, but without sufficient depth of information, they take on a life of their own. In so many respects, the drive to destigmatise mental illness is wonderful and important. But it has had an unintended side effect: it's triggered a chain reaction of misinformation that complicates the very topic we're trying to understand.

Collateral damage

The first step in this chain reaction is that the goalposts that define what counts as mental illness are being picked up and moved. In the rush to destigmatise mental illness, and the confusion about what it really is, all kinds of normal negative emotions and experiences are being labelled as mental disorders – or at the very least, as problems that need to be instantly fixed. Take, for example, anxiety disorders. On Twitter recently, a professor in the States complained that many of his students were asking to be excused from giving oral presentations on the grounds of anxiety. Of course they should be anxious, he tweeted, they're doing a presentation. There was a considerable backlash against this, with many people arguing that students with anxiety disorders shouldn't be forced to give presentations, and he deleted the tweet.

His attitude seemed callous, but I could relate to the dilemma he faced. In one of the modules I taught as a lecturer, students were required to give presentations. When some of them asked to be excused from doing so because they were anxious, it was hard to know the right thing to do. It's wrong, of course, to force someone in the throes of an anxiety disorder to give a presentation, particularly those with social anxiety disorder, which is defined by an intense and debilitating fear of how others judge you. Making these individuals present in front of their classmates is akin to forcing someone with a spider phobia to hold a tarantula, or trapping someone with claustrophobia in a lift. It's cruel, and the course assessment for these students should be adjusted. In fact, there was a devastating case in 2018 of a UK university student, Natasha Abrahart, who took her own life on the day she was due to give a big presentation. There are many contributing factors that lead to suicide, but one element in this case was that Natasha had social anxiety disorder, and she wasn't able to get any adjustments to the assessment. Missing it would have meant failing the module, and the course – something she would have experienced, her mother said at the inquest, as a 'huge failure'.[5]

This story makes my blood run cold. But the difficulty is that many students who are anxious about presentations do not have an anxiety *disorder* like Natasha's. I'm not saying their concerns aren't real, or that these milder problems don't need addressing. I'm saying that this kind of anxiety is not the same as the clinical version, and shouldn't be treated as such. In fact, for many milder forms of anxiety, excusing students from giving the presentation would be totally unhelpful: one of the main ways in which anxiety is maintained is by avoidance. If someone who feels a bit anxious about giving a presentation never does so, then they can never find out what it's actually like and thus discover that perhaps it isn't as bad as they fear or at the least learn ways to cope – two key ways of reducing future anxiety. The problem is that it's very difficult for lecturers to know which students really do need alternative assessments and which students just need support and encouragement. Since we've started talking publicly about mental health, the language people are using to describe common, transient negative feelings has become caught up in the language we should be reserving for mental illness. Maintaining a distinction between the two – which is essential if we are to effectively help those on both sides – is vital.

The infinite challenge of defining mental illness

The truth is, the professionals *themselves* keep moving the goalposts. Determining what mental illness is turns out to be a tricky, fallible, ever-changing process. As we'll see, every few years, the official guidelines for diagnosing mental disorders are published, and every time there are changes: adjustments for where the authors think normal experience ends and pathology begins. Even among the experts there is confusion, debate and disagreement over what counts as mental illness – and even, as I've said, whether the terms 'illness' or 'disorder' should ever be used when describing psychological distress.

This, I argue, is partly why those destigmatising campaigns have inadvertently led to misinformation about mental illness. The confusion is no longer exclusively behind closed academic doors: it's in the public domain now too. It can hardly be any wonder that as vague, complex and sometimes conflicting information makes its way into the public consciousness, people start making up their own minds about where those lines are drawn. In the absence of clear-cut rules and advice, it is understandable that we might start couching many of our own experiences in these psychiatric terms – unlike previous generations, for example, today's students have actually heard of anxiety disorders.

It is not in any way my intention to dismiss or belittle the campaigning efforts to increase awareness of and openness about mental illness. It's wonderful that this public conversation has begun, it really is. It's brave and impressive that people with mental illness have discussed their experiences. Writing this book, and debating how much of my own story to include, has given me renewed respect for the people who have been so frank and honest about their darkest days. People who have talked and written openly about their most private fears, their vulnerability, their loneliness – these pioneers made me and so many others realise we're not alone, and that getting better is possible. Every person who speaks out, every article that's written, is one tiny step forward, one extra whisper that it's okay to admit you've experienced it too. I'm not for one second suggesting that people shouldn't have done this, or that they should ever stop.

On the contrary. Right now, there are still thousands and thousands of individuals reluctant to admit that they have a mental illness, aware of the very real stigma they would face if they opened their mouths. In fact, a 2020 study investigated why UK adolescents aged ten to nineteen don't seek help for mental health problems, and the number one cited reason was stigma.[6] Other reasons given were negative attitudes towards mental health services and professionals, and poor mental health literacy (i.e. a poor understanding of mental disorders and the possible help available). And this was among young people, the group who are supposedly most attuned to their mental health. 'Teens who are most in need of mental health attention are reluctant to seek help,' the authors concluded. So the conversation has started, and that's brilliant, but we still have such a long way to go.

An epidemic of mental illness?

To progress the conversation, we first need to understand whether rates of mental illness are higher today than in the past, especially among young people. The arrival of Covid-19 certainly added to these concerns, and we'll explore the possible effect of the pandemic later in this book, but this sense of a new, accelerating mental health crisis was prevalent long before the virus appeared and it dominates the mental health conversation. In September 2016, for example, the television programme *This Morning* ran a piece entitled 'Anxiety: The mental health epidemic sweeping Britain'. In September 2018, the *Guardian* published an article with the headline 'Mental health issues in young people up sixfold in England since 1995'.[7] In January 2020, the *New York Times* published the article 'Why are young Americans killing themselves?' which began: 'Teenagers and young adults in the United States are being ravaged by a mental health crisis – and we are doing nothing about it.'[8] The notion of a new epidemic of mental illness has become widely accepted on both sides of the Atlantic.

In this book, we will examine the data behind these headlines, and we will also explore the many factors that might contribute to these changing rates. Because along with concerns about things getting worse, there has been a great deal of attention on *why* that might be. What is it about this generation, about today's society, we wonder, that could mean we're suddenly in a collective psychiatric crisis?

A host of explanations have been put forward, largely focusing on young people, as this is where the possible increase seems to be happening. I will examine many of these theories in this book: the idea that we have somehow raised a generation of 'snowflakes', less able to cope with life's challenges compared to previous generations; the alternative possibility that today's young people are growing up in a legitimately more stressful, uncertain world (even pre-Covid) than that of their forebears; and perhaps the most prevalent explanation: social media. These are all legitimate theories, all more complex than they might first seem, and they deserve our attention. But in many ways, this question – of *why* we might have increased rates of mental illness – is a red herring. It's not where we should be focusing our energy – certainly not all of it.

We also need to be asking the bigger, age-old questions: what *is* mental illness? What causes it, and what can we do about it? Across generations, there has always been a minority of individuals who have become seriously psychologically unwell, and the causes run deeper than any fresh crisis or fad. I'm very interested in what precisely is happening in today's society – and begin with a brief analysis of the evidence for a new wave of mental illness. But this book also seeks to answer the bigger and, in my view, far more important question of what mental illness is and always has been. Understanding this will help us understand whether the current 'epidemic' is a real one or whether something else is going on, and what exactly that might be.

What we need above all is clarity. For all the ambiguity and uncertainty, there's a lot we do know about mental illness, and that's what this book is about too. For example, we know that the vast majority of people who will ever develop a mental disorder will have it by their early twenties, and I'll explain why adolescence is such a period of risk. I'll talk about causes: why it is that some people can become unwell in the absence of any obvious external stress, while others are simply impermeable to mental illness, no matter what life throws at them, no matter how harrowing their experiences. I'll tell you how we go about treating mental illness, the therapy and medication, and talk about recovery, about why the term 'recovery' is itself controversial. And lastly, I'll stand on top of the hill and look into the horizon, and think about what needs to happen next: a better approach to talking about mental distress and illness, and how to support ourselves and each other.

As we develop our understanding of what mental illness actually is, we must also recognise what it *isn't*. Sadness and stress and worry are part of the human condition. The medicalisation of what should be considered normal and the categorising of all suffering as a disorder helps no one. This book is about mental illness, but it's about the other end of the spectrum too: a rallying cry that psychological pain has always existed, and that there are ways of talking about it without calling everyone unwell.

CHAPTER 1

Rising rates

Between 2008 and 2018, prescriptions for antidepressant medications in the UK increased from 36 million to 70.9 million.[1] A study of twenty-nine countries – including Australia, Canada and many in Europe – found that all of them had seen an increase in antidepressant prescriptions between 2000 and 2015, doubling on average.[2] Antidepressants are used to treat many disorders, including depression, OCD and anxiety disorders, so if more people are taking them now than in the past, this could be an indication that mental illness is on the up. By this metric, the number of people with mental illness has exploded.

But of course there are other possible explanations for the rise in prescriptions. It could be that thanks to increased public awareness and the drive to destigmatise mental illness, people are more willing to seek help when their distress becomes unmanageable. This would be a wholly good thing. It could also be that GPs and other prescribers are getting better at identifying and diagnosing genuine cases of mental illness – again, a good thing. Alternatively, prescriptions might be increasing because some doctors are overprescribing: handing out prescriptions too readily for milder problems, or prescribing because of a lack of available alternatives like talking therapy. All of these could be true at the same time.

If we want to know whether rates of mental illness are genuinely increasing, then ideally we don't want to rely only on data from people who are already seeking help. A far better option is to measure the prevalence of symptoms in the general population and see if those have increased. In contrast to 'clinical' samples, in which the participants being measured are already seeking or getting help, 'community' samples are composed of a representative group of people from across society: a range of ages, genders and ethnicities, for example. Unless people with mental illness diagnoses are actively screened and excluded from the study, and assuming the community sample is large enough, it should provide an illustrative snapshot of the population as a whole, containing people who fall across the full spectrum of mental health and illness.

Studies that take this approach use two main methods to assess symptoms: self-report questionnaires and interviews. Self-report questionnaires are quick and easy to use, so can be distributed to large groups of participants. They present people with a list of symptoms, like 'I felt down about myself' or 'Someone was controlling my thoughts', and the respondent then decides how much they have experienced that symptom over a set period of time – the last two weeks, say, or the last six months – usually by selecting from a limited range of possible answers, such as a five-point scale from 'Strongly agree' to 'Strongly disagree'.

There are many well-established, robust questionnaires that measure symptoms of mental illness, and they cover all different disorders. For example, a thirteen-item questionnaire called the Short Mood and Feelings Questionnaire (SMFQ) was developed in 1995 as a brief measure of depressive symptoms in children and adolescents.[3] Respondents read statements such as 'I didn't enjoy anything at all', 'I was a bad person' and 'I felt lonely' and answer whether each item applied to them over the preceding two weeks using a three-point scale: Not True (0), Sometimes (1), or True (2).

The important thing to remember about self-report questionnaires is that they are not designed to be definitive measures of a disorder. As we will see, context is important when it comes to understanding mental health symptoms, and there's no context at all when it comes to answers on a questionnaire. For example, someone could score relatively highly on a depression measure if they've recently received some bad news or gone through a big life change, but it doesn't mean they're clinically depressed. Instead, researchers try to choose a cut-off score that indicates a person *might* be depressed – those who use the SMFQ, for example, often use a threshold of twelve or above to indicate possible mental illness[4] – but they warn that this isn't clear-cut. The creators of the SMFQ specifically state that such measures 'might better be regarded as 'nets' than as screens ... [they] will miss a number of cases of interest and pick up a good deal of other material'. In other words, a high score on a measure like the SMFQ is a useful indicator that you might want to assess someone further for potential depression, but in and of itself, it's not a measure of the disorder.

This detail often gets lost though. Consider a study reported in a 2017 *Guardian* article under the headline 'One in four girls have depression by the time they hit 14'.[5] This was a population-based study in which more than 11,000 young people completed the SMFQ. The researchers found that 24% of fourteen-year-old girls scored at or above the cut-off score of twelve – the figure that made the headline – as did 9% of boys. But from a self-report questionnaire alone, we can't know for sure how many of these young people really had depression. What the study actually showed was that one in four girls reported a reasonably high number of negative feelings in the previous two weeks, like feeling tired or lonely or down about themselves. That's bad, for sure – but we have to be very careful about equating this with a depressive disorder.

One way round this issue is to use clinical interviews. These are similar to questionnaires, in that they ask the person about a series of symptoms. However, they are often considered superior to and more reliable than questionnaires as they are conducted by a trained professional and allow the opportunity for the interviewer to ask follow-up questions about severity and duration of symptoms. But bear in mind they're not perfect either: they're more costly and time-consuming to administer, generally meaning that fewer participants can be included. Also, the interviewers aren't necessarily *clinically* trained. US psychiatrist Allen Frances – who has helped devise guidelines for what counts as a mental disorder – has expressed concern about the impact of this. In fact, he says this issue means the oft-quoted 'one in four' stat is probably an overestimate:

> Never believe the extremely high rates of mental disorders routinely reported by epidemiological studies in psychiatry – usually labelling about 25% of the general population as mentally ill in the past year ... Phone surveys are done by non-clinicians following a highly structured format that allows no clinical judgment whether the symptoms reported cause sufficient clinically significant distress and impairment to qualify as a mental disorder ... The rates reported in studies are really only upper limits, not accurate approximations of true rates. They should be, but never are, reported as such.[6]

Both questionnaires and interviews are therefore likely overestimates, and only ever give an *indication* of a disorder, but assuming the same specific questionnaire or interview is used throughout the time period being examined, they are the best we have and better than relying on the number of people seeking help from their doctor. So, bearing in mind all of these qualifications, does the data suggest that rates of mental illness are increasing?

The evidence

In 2012, the psychologist and sociologist Joan Busfield published a paper examining exactly this question.[7] In it, she reviewed lots of studies that used self-report questionnaires and clinical interviews to measure mental illness at different points in time, the earliest dating from 1952 and the most recent from

2007. There was a mix of results, with some finding an increase in rates, and some finding rates were stable. However, based on the best-quality studies, the evidence was in favour of the latter: no significant change in rates of mental illness in the time period up to 2007. This is how she summarised her findings:

> The claims [of increased mental illness and decreased mental well-being] are based on weak foundations. While there is some evidence to support such claims, equally there is plenty of evidence that does not. Indeed, when the same or similar structured diagnostic instruments and similar diagnostic criteria are used to measure the same disorders ... the comparison indicates that mental illness has not been increasing over the longer term.

Interesting stuff – but this only takes us up to 2007. It's perfectly possible that rates didn't increase back then, but that there's been a shift more recently.

In 2019, a meta-analysis led by sociologist Dirk Richter looked at data from forty-two studies from all over the world – mainly Western Europe and North America, but also Asia, South America and Australia.[8] There was a combined sample size of 1,035,697 adult participants, and the studies used either self-report questionnaires, clinical interviews, or both. Some measured specific disorders: anxiety disorders, substance abuse or depression; others measured what the meta-analysis authors called 'psychological distress', a broader concept essentially covering both anxiety and depressive symptoms. In all forty-two studies, data was collected at two different time points, between two and twenty-nine years apart. The earliest was 1978, and the latest was 2015. They found that, averaged across all forty-two studies, there was a statistically significant increase in these types of mental illness and mental distress across time, but it was 'small'. They note that this finding is 'obviously at odds with the evidence of a tremendous increase in mental healthcare utilization' and also with the 'public impression of a mental health epidemic during the same period'.

There is evidence of a similar rise in mental disorders in adolescents. One UK study, led by the NHS, used clinical interviews with approximately 9,000 five-to-fifteen-year-olds, carried out in 1999, 2004 and 2017. The interviews covered lots of different potential diagnoses: depression and anxiety disorders, but also others like conduct disorder (characterised by antisocial behaviour), hyperactivity disorders like ADHD and eating disorders. The authors found a 'slight increase' in overall rates of depression and anxiety disorders from 1999 to 2017, while the prevalence of other disorders remained constant. In 1999, 9.7% of five-to-fifteen-year-olds had a diagnosable disorder; in 2004, this figure increased to 10.1%; and in 2017 it was 11.2%. So again, we see a similar story: there is evidence of an increased prevalence of mental illness, but the increase is relatively small. Tamsin Ford, a child psychiatrist who developed the survey, said: 'It was smaller than we thought ... It's not huge, not the epidemic you see reported.'[9]

Self-harm

One of our most fundamental biological drives, one we share with all other animals, is the desire to avoid pain. We're wary of trying risky activities in case we injure ourselves and we learn very quickly to avoid things that hurt us. Our aversion to pain is ancient, and makes perfect evolutionary sense: we avoid pain to keep ourselves safe. And yet, a significant minority of people behave in ways that fly directly in the face of this. Some people deliberately injure themselves, most usually by cutting the skin with a blade, but sometimes by other means like burning or hitting themselves. This is self-harm: the deliberate, intentional act of damaging your own body tissue. There is considerable current concern about an increase in these behaviours in particular, since they may be an indication of increased rates of mental distress and illness. So what exactly is the relationship here, and what does the data show about changing rates?

Most commonly, people self-harm because they feel over-whelming negative emotions, like sadness or guilt or shame. Pain is highly distracting, so the sensation helps to shift focus away from these intensely distressing thoughts and feelings. You might suppose that perhaps people who self-harm don't feel physical pain as much as others do, which is why they are able to harm themselves, but the evidence to date suggests they are perfectly able to feel pain.[10] In fact, many people self-harm *because* it's painful, because of its power to distract. In the words of psychiatrist Bessel van der Kolk, people cut themselves 'to replace overwhelming emotions with definable sensations'.[11] The desire to escape their negative emotions is so great that the physical pain seems a price worth paying. In short, people self-harm as a form of emotion regulation. As we shall see later in the book, this is a process that's developing in adolescence, and one that is disrupted pretty much across the board in many different mental disorders.

Some people self-harm for a slightly different reason – which might run in parallel with the above: they feel they *deserve* to be in pain. As we'll see, your feelings towards yourself are an important part of many mental illnesses. A hallmark of depression, for example, is a feeling of worthlessness. People with depression don't tend to like themselves. Other disorders, particularly eating disorders, often involve low levels of self-worth and high levels of self-criticism. Once a person dislikes or hates themselves, the idea of hurting themselves no longer seems so foreign. One study, for example, showed that people with high levels of self-criticism are able to endure pain for longer than those with low levels.[12] Self-injury becomes a way of meting out a punishment they feel they deserve – for errors they feel they've made, or feelings or thoughts rising think they shouldn't experience. As Sian Bradley, a mental health campaigner, explained on an MQ Open Mind podcast:

It's quite dangerous to just always assume that it's because somebody might want to end their life, because I do think quite often [self-harm and suicide] are very separate. It's always just been a way to ... deal with these overwhelming emotions, to punish myself for imaginary crimes that I've done, for failures, for things like that. It's not been anything related to wanting to end my life at all, it's just been something to deal with the pain right now.[13]

It's important to note that some people who self-harm once will rarely or never do so again, and some cause themselves only superficial injury (such as repeatedly scratching their skin). But for others, self-harm becomes chronic and severe – sometimes requiring hospital treatment – and is the only way they can find to cope with their feelings. This is why the oft-thrown criticism of people self-harming 'to get attention' seems odd to me. People who self-harm are intensely distressed, and if that happens to be noticed – as a side effect – well, that's good. They need to be noticed; they need support and help.

There is some ongoing debate about whether frequent and severe self-harm should be a mental illness in and of itself. But what we do know is that in people who have a mental illness, self-harm often appears. The exact number varies a lot between studies, but somewhere in the region of 30–82% of individuals with a mental disorder have self-harmed.[14] It was once considered to be largely tied to borderline personality disorder, a disorder characterised by poor emotion regulation and problems with social relationships. But it's actually a *transdiagnostic* phenomenon, appearing in depression, anxiety disorders, OCD, post-traumatic stress disorder, eating disorders and substance use disorders, among others. In addition, even though the goal of self-harm is specifically *not* suicide (as Bradley says), people who self-harm are at increased risk of later suicide attempts. This all suggests that there is some relationship between self-harm and mental distress and disorder, which makes intuitive sense, particularly when this behaviour is chronic and severe.

To return to our original question: the best available research suggests rates of self-harm are increasing in our society. One study compared rates of self-harm among fourteen-year-olds in 2005 and 2015.[15] In 2005, the teenagers were asked whether they had *ever* tried to harm or kill themselves: 11.8% said yes. The 2015 group were asked a slightly different question (because the groups came from two different cohort studies): whether they had hurt themselves on purpose in any way *in the past year*. Because of the narrower parameter, you might expect fewer teenagers to have answered yes in 2015, all other things being equal. In fact 14.5% said yes.

Another study conducted clinical interviews with a large group of sixteen-to-seventy-four-year-olds in England in 2000, 2007 and 2014.[16] At each time point, between 6,000 and 7,000 people were interviewed. Across the whole dataset, the researchers found that the number of people who reported ever engaging in self-harm (across their lifetime) increased from 2.4% in 2000 to 6.4% in 2014. The biggest increase was amongst females aged sixteen to twenty-four, whose levels of self-harm increased from 6.5% in 2000 to 19.7% in 2014. This is a really big jump, and one we need to consider carefully later in this book, when we think about *why* these rates might be increasing.

Increase in suicides

'Killing oneself is, anyway, a misnomer. We don't kill ourselves. We are simply defeated by the long, hard struggle to stay alive.' So wrote Sally Brampton in her memoir about depression, *Shoot the Damn Dog*, published in 2008.[17] I read it that year, in the months before I became unwell. When my depression hit, I wished I hadn't. The book captures astutely the aching awfulness of depression, and her description of just how bad things could become haunted me. (This is why I generally don't recommend memoirs of mental illness for people who are in the depths of it themselves – they are more useful for friends and families, to understand, or for when those who suffer are feeling better.) It's ultimately a hopeful book – it's about Brampton making sense of her depression and suicidal thoughts, and her gradual recovery. So my heart sank when, by chance, I read an article in 2016 saying she had died. She had taken her own life.

Around 800,000 people across the world take their own life each year.[18] Brampton's book stuck with me because it captures so well what suicide is about: it's not about wanting to die, she wrote, so much as 'a fervent wish not to go on living'. People die by suicide when they feel they can no longer stay alive. Sometimes people's lives become sufficiently painful and difficult that they take their own lives in the absence of any diagnosable mental disorder, but most of the time they do have one. (The exact percentage is hard to ascertain. It is often quoted that around 90% of people who kill themselves had a mental disorder,[19] but this figure is reached from 'psychological autopsies', which include interviewing family members about the deceased person to try and understand the contributing factors. It's possible that, in the wake of a suicide, family members are particularly primed to look for signs of preceding mental illness.)

Globally, suicide rates are decreasing. Data from the Global Burden of Disease Study in 2016 showed that, when you combine information from sixty-three countries, rates dropped by a third between 1990 and 2016.[20] This seems mostly to be driven by considerable declines in suicide in China and India – and these drops could be because of a host of reasons: economic growth, urbanisation, better standards of living, improved access to medical care and restricted access to certain methods of suicide. Around 80% of suicides occur in low-and middle-income countries, so these changes in quality of life make an important difference to worldwide rates.[21] However, the concern is that, in the West, rates are actually increasing.

In 2019, the Office for National Statistics released data about suicides in the UK in 2018. When everyone is grouped together (age and sex), it showed there was a small but significant increase from the previous year: there were 10.1 suicides per 100,000 population in 2017, and 11.2 suicides per

100,000 population in 2018. These rates followed several years of decline, matching levels not seen since 2013. A single-year increase like this shouldn't immediately trigger alarm bells – the official report from the ONS said: 'Suicide rates tend to fluctuate on a year-to-year basis. It is therefore too early to say whether the latest increase represents a change in the recent trend.'[22]

When we break things down by age and sex, however, something more concerning emerges. In females aged ten to twenty-four, the suicide rate has steadily increased for several years, from 1.8 deaths per 100,000 females in 2012 to 3.3 deaths per 100,000 in 2018. The collective attention about suicide is usually focused on males, as they make up 75% of suicide deaths (possibly because males experiencing psychological distress are less likely to seek help, so things escalate for them). But this data, combined with the self-harm data, suggests that something might be shifting in adolescent females. In the United States, meanwhile, data released in 2018 from the National Center for Health Statistics showed that, between 1999 and 2017, the rate of suicide has increased among both males and females, across all age groups.[23] Among ten-to-twenty-four-year-olds specifically, the rate of suicide per 100,000 has increased from 3.5 to 7.5 in females and from 18.7 to 26 in males. The absolute numbers are small, of course – it is exceptionally rare for a young person to take their own life – but each one of these individuals represents a permanent and aching absence in a family, a friendship group, a community – a real person in distress who didn't get the help they badly needed. Understanding what might account for these rises, as we do later in this book, is important work.

Impact of a pandemic

Everything in this chapter so far has taken us up to around 2018. But of course, since then, there has been a global, monumental change. Almost as soon as Covid-19 took hold, there was a wave of concern about how it might increase rates of mental illness and suicide. The full effects of the pandemic will not be known for some time, and the slow cycle of research will also delay our understanding, but the urgency of the situation has expedited things a bit: there's been an enormous effort to collect and share data already. Perhaps unsurprisingly, this data indicates that Covid-19 is having a notable impact on our psychological well-being.

In October 2020, a group of UK researchers published a study about the mental health effects of the first month of lockdown. They were able to make use of an existing, ongoing study: the UK Household Longitudinal Study, which started in 2009 and regularly collected interview data from participants.[24] In April 2020, over 17,000 participants aged 16 to 80 completed an extra survey, relating to Covid-19. They answered questions about their financial situation over the last two months and also filled in the General Health Questionnaire-12 (GHQ-12). This is a frequently used measure of 'mental health, distress and well-being' that determines how often the respondent has recently experienced twelve particular symptoms. The questions include 'Have you lost much sleep over worry?', 'Have you been able to enjoy your normal day-to-day activities?' and 'Have you been feeling happy, all things considered?' For each question, there are four options (slightly tweaked depending on the question): Not at all (0 points), No more than usual (1), Rather more than usual (2) and Much more than usual (3). This is clearly not an in-depth measure of any specific disorder, but it is a quick broad-brush measure of distress that can be a screening tool for diagnosable disorders.

In the previous year, the group's mean score on the GHQ-12 was 11.5 (out of a maximum score of 36); in April 2020 it was 12.6, a statistically significant increase. The researchers also calculated how many people were considered to have 'clinically significant levels of mental distress'. To do this, they gave participants zero points for either of the first two answers (Not at all, No more than usual) and one point for either of the more affirmative answers (Rather more than usual, Much more than usual). This meant that, as a twelve-item questionnaire, the maximum score, indicating maximum distress, would be 12. The researchers used a threshold of 4 or above, as others have done, to indicate a clinically significant level of distress. Across the previous year, 18.9% of people met this threshold; in April 2020, it was 27.3%.

The director of the Institute for Fiscal Studies, Paul Johnson, tweeted about the findings from their first study in June 2020, when they were shared as part of a working paper, writing: 'The mental health consequences of lockdown have been severe … This is a big, widespread and swift deterioration.' And yet, it would have been more surprising if we *hadn't* seen increases in people's distress and unhappiness around April 2020. The GHQ-12 questions include items about feeling under strain, feeling like you're not playing a useful role in society, and feeling unable to concentrate. It's understandable that more people said yes to those things right at the start of a global pandemic. When that data was collected, everything had suddenly changed and losses were recent and acute. These initial numbers need to be interpreted with caution: psychological distress in response to temporary stress and disruption is normal, and not necessarily an indicator of mental illness.

The trouble is that the lockdown of spring 2020 was not a one-off but the start of a prolonged period of disruption. Dirk Richter, who has been studying changing rates of mental illness for twenty years, says the long-term nature of the pandemic is critical. In October 2020, he said: 'The data from earlier recessions, for example, very clearly say that the long-term fallout will be much more important, in terms of suicide rates, than what happened during the height of the distress. As long as there was no second wave, I was optimistic. But now I think things are really going down.'[25]

It was also evident almost immediately that some people have been hit far harder by the pandemic than others. In the above study, the increases in GHQ-12 scores were highest for eighteen-to-thirty-four-year-olds, women, and people living with young children. They were also higher for people who were employed before the pandemic, compared to those who were already unemployed – presumably because these people experienced a bigger shift in their daily life, included potential job losses.

For another study, over 12,000 adults were interviewed weekly for the first three weeks of lockdown (25 March to 14 April 2020).[26] The participants were asked whether they had experienced any of ten 'adversities'. Some were financial (e.g. whether the participant or their partner had lost their job), some were related to basic needs (e.g. whether they had lost their accommodation or were unable to access sufficient food), and some were directly related to the virus (e.g. whether the participant had Covid-19 or somebody close to them was hospitalised or had died). In week three, for example, 16.7% reported a major loss in household income and 3.5% the loss of someone close to them. Most pertinently, the relative risk of experiencing these adversities correlated with the participant's socio-economic position (SEP) – a combined measure of education level, household income, employment and housing status. Those with the lowest SEP experienced the highest number of adverse events, and were especially likely to experience financial hardship and difficulty accessing basic needs (food, medication and accommodation).

This is important because, as we shall see later in the book, stressful events and socio-economic hardship are – for everyone – key factors that increase the risk of mental illness. For this reason, if some demographics are more likely to experience stress and disruption from the pandemic, they might be more at risk of developing a resultant mental disorder. For example, there is some initial evidence, from a separate report, that the mental health of people from BAME groups has been more adversely affected by the pandemic than that of white people.[27] Two contributing factors to this could be the disproportionate number of Covid-19 infections and deaths among BAME communities, and the increased risk that

BAME individuals will experience the economic adversities described above.

All this will need to be investigated in more depth in the coming months and years, not least because BAME is a broad umbrella term that may miss meaningful differences between specific ethnic groups. But what this does all indicate is that, for those who are facing existing or new economic disadvantage, the pandemic and its consequences could be the 'trigger' for serious psychological difficulty over the long term. This certainly doesn't mean everyone who has been stressed in 2020 will develop a mental illness: as we will later see, the majority of people who experience trauma and stressful life events navigate them without developing a disorder. But we need to bear in mind that stress increases risk, and that there has been no shortage of stressful events in this pandemic.

Routes to specific mental disorders

There are also potential direct mental health consequences of actually having the virus, or looking after those who do. There have been predictions of an increase in post-traumatic stress in both Covid-19 survivors[28] and healthcare workers,[29] with one research group referring to PTSD as the potential 'second tsunami' of the pandemic.[30] There are also predictions – again of a 'tsunami'[31] – of cases of post-viral depression, a variant of mental disorder seen after other pandemics such as SARS in 2003 and the Spanish Flu in 1918. But I would be cautious about these predictions and their provocative language until the hard data comes in.

There are other, more specific elements of this global event that could impact people's mental health. It would be reasonable to predict, for instance, that people with sanitation- and contamination-based OCD – who have obsessive fears about germs and cleanliness – could be badly affected. Thorough handwashing has been essential to tackling the virus, and was widely promoted everywhere. To ensure we washed them thoroughly enough, the government even advised we sing 'Happy Birthday' twice while doing so. This was a nightmare for people who already washed their hands obsessively and to the point of pain and skin damage. In March 2020, writer David Adam – who himself has OCD – wrote: 'For some people with obsessive–compulsive disorder ... to be warned they must scrub to protect themselves from an invisible enemy, and to do so in a ritualistic way with internal musical accompaniment, is akin to inviting a demon to come for tea. Some of these people have spent years trying not to wash their hands, often as a prescribed part of their treatment.'[32]

For many people with this type of OCD, the pandemic could have triggered an unravelling of many years of dedicated therapeutic work. For others, the stress of the pandemic and its focus on sanitation could be a 'trigger' that sets off new cases of this disorder in people who were already vulnerable to it. Again, there are relevant lessons from other pandemics, in which increased cases of OCD have been documented six to twelve months after the outbreak. In June 2020, the psychiatrist Debanjan Banerjee wrote: 'Whenever the strategies against an infection involve repetitive behaviours, it carries the risk of increasing obsessional disorders. It might not be evident in the active phase of the outbreak due to under-detection, disruption of medical services and alternate public health priorities.'[33]

And then, of course, there is the social side of the pandemic. For people prone to social anxiety disorder or agoraphobia – characterised by fear of being in public places or simply being outside the home – the idea of meeting up with people, paired with the fear of catching the virus (or unwittingly giving it to someone), could be incredibly difficult after months at home. In addition, a huge number of people, with or without an existing mental disorder, will have experienced prolonged social isolation and loneliness – and it is well established that this can cause and exacerbate mental illness.

For all these reasons it is entirely reasonable that we're concerned about the effects of Covid-19 on our mental health, but it is simply too early to know what they will be. We will have to wait and see what the data says in time. But we must not let the arrival of the pandemic cloud the fact that this concern about rapidly rising rates of mental illness existed long before the coronavirus reared its head. And while the evidence surveyed in this chapter suggests that rates were and are on the up, with the most noticeable and concerning rise being that of self-harm in adolescent girls, the extent of much of the increase was not as grave as many reports would have us think. We may yet face an increase in mental illness, brought on by the pandemic, but before that, we were not experiencing the crisis we might have thought. Rather, as I hope to show over the course of this book, something more subtle was – and is – taking place. But to understand what that is, we must first attempt to understand what is actually meant by the term 'mental illness', which turns out to be a complex and changeable business.

CHAPTER 2

On a continuum

Scientists must simplify and categorise the world in order to understand it. Typically, psychologists help us understand human experience by separating it into three broad categories: thoughts, feelings and behaviours. These three pillars interact with and influence each other: our mood affects the way we think, our thoughts affect the way we behave, our actions affect our mood and so on. In fact, in a new patient's first appointment, many cognitive behavioural therapists – a common type of therapy, prescribed by the NHS – will write down these three categories on a piece of paper as the three points of a triangle, drawing double-ended arrows between them to illustrate their relationship.

We all think, feel and do a thousand different things every day. But while these thoughts, feelings and behaviours vary, we are fundamentally creatures of habit, and we tend to get into patterns with all three. When any of these patterns become extreme – if we consistently think bizarre thoughts or feel miserable or act aggressively towards others, for example – they can cause us problems. To use a simple definition: when these extreme patterns become uncontrollable and affect our ability to live the life we want, then we have moved into the realm of what many people might want to call 'mental illness'.

Except that, of course, it's not that simple. After all, how do we decide at what point something becomes sufficiently 'extreme' to be considered a symptom of mental illness? The fundamental problem is that the symptoms of mental illness lie on a *continuum* with the emotions, thoughts and behaviours that healthy people experience all the time in their daily lives, and these smooth continua make it really difficult to pin down the cut-off point at which a negative experience or mental health problem becomes a symptom of mental illness. Part of the challenge of defining mental illness, therefore, is the challenge of deciding where to locate these cut-off points.

Why we need cut-off points

You may be wondering why we need to create cut-off points at all. Can't we just accept that there is a seamless continuum between normal and pathological experiences, and leave it at that? In fact, many mental health professionals – particularly psychotherapists and psychologists – are not especially interested in identifying whether someone meets some predetermined threshold or what exactly their diagnosis might be. Instead, these clinicians are more interested in whether the person is experiencing symptoms that are causing them distress, or affecting their ability to function in their life. And some researchers are now campaigning to view mental illness as matters of degree, shades of a problem, rather than entirely discrete categories. But though they may be artificial, thresholds and diagnostic labels are still widely used because they can be very useful, and for certain practical purposes they are essential.

Most obviously we need to be able to decide who has a specific disorder and who doesn't for some treatment purposes: it's not practical or safe to offer antidepressants to everyone who reports being unhappy, for example, so ideally we need cut-off points so that clinicians have standardised guidelines about when to prescribe medication. Such guidelines are crucial for consistency, safety and fairness across a health service. In countries like the US, these boundaries are also important because they allow people to access insurance payments: you need to meet diagnostic criteria before treatment will be offered or covered.

Cut-offs are also essential in research into the effectiveness of treatments. If researchers want to evaluate the effectiveness of cognitive behavioural therapy (CBT) for those who suffer from panic disorder, for example, they need a group of patients who adhere to a shared definition of panic disorder and exhibit similar symptoms: in other words, a group that all score above a widely agreed threshold on a diagnostic test for panic disorder. Without that shared understanding, the research is useless – both to other researchers and to doctors attempting to treat patients with panic disorder.

Finally, cut-off points are useful because they allow both clinicians and researchers to say who has improved after treatment. If a researcher develops a new type of psychological therapy and wants to test its effectiveness on a hundred people with depression, then she will want to know how many people no longer have depression at the end of the course of treatment. To do that, she needs to have a definitive threshold that marks the difference between depressed and non-depressed. Similarly, a doctor who prescribes a patient with antidepressants will need to assess whether the patient is still depressed after several months on the medication.

For all these reasons, even though they are artificial, we continue to draw distinct lines between mental health and illness – because we have to. But as we will see, paradoxically, the more precise a cut-off point is, the more arbitrary it is, whereas the vaguer it is, the more accurately it reflects reality. So how do the experts go about it?

Two examples of continua

There are many different symptoms of depression, but low mood is one of the core, most common symptoms. Like pretty much every other psychological phenomenon, low mood exists on a spectrum. Imagine a line marked 0 at one end and 100 at the other. Think of 0 as a very happy, upbeat mood: a strong sense of gratitude, optimism and contentment. Now think of 100 as the worst mood possible: a dark, inescapable sense of utter hopelessness. Now consider numbers 1–99, each point a gradually changing degree of mood, from very happy to desperately sad. At which number would you say someone is experiencing a symptom of depression, rather than just an everyday low mood? 65, perhaps? Let's say for the sake of argument we could agree a cut-off point at 65 – then what about someone at 64? Is a low mood of 64/100 meaningfully different to a 65/100? And bear in mind that in reality there aren't just one hundred shades of mood – there are many hundreds or even thousands.

As we will see below, a diagnosis of depression is never reached on the basis of low mood alone, so this illustration is somewhat academic. In reality, depression involves many symptoms, and a certain number of them must be present before a diagnosis of depression will be considered. But all of them share this same issue: that there is no clear boundary for when any depressive symptom has moved from the realm of 'normal experience' to become a sure-fire sign of a disorder.

It is intuitively understandable that a common symptom like low mood exists on a continuum, but what about symptoms of psychosis? The word 'psychosis' is poorly understood – it's often inaccurately used to describe someone extremely angry or violent (e.g. 'my psychotic ex-girlfriend'), but that's not what it means. (It's also not the same thing as 'psychopathic': psychopathy is a personality disorder characterised by a persistent lack of empathy and guilt, a flat emotional experience, and manipulative and harmful behaviour towards others.) Instead, psychosis is often characterised as 'a loss of contact with reality', and the two key symptoms are delusions (very simply – believing things that aren't real) and hallucinations (experiencing things that aren't real). Psychotic symptoms can be triggered by certain drugs, medical conditions or extreme stress, but they also appear in several mental disorders, most notably schizophrenia and bipolar disorder. You might think that cut-off points are much easier to decide with these sort of symptoms. Is that the case?

To answer this question, we will need to be more specific in our definitions. Delusions are extreme beliefs that are held despite overwhelming evidence to demonstrate that they are not true, and they often involve themes of paranoia (like 'government spies are tracking my every move'), or grandiosity (like believing you are God). Hallucinations are sensory experiences not grounded in reality: auditory verbal hallucinations – hearing voices in your head – are common among those with psychosis, but some experience visual hallucinations too – seeing people and images that aren't there. There are also hallucinations in other senses: tasting or smelling things that aren't there, or feeling things like the sensation of insects crawling on your skin. Such delusions and hallucinations can be brought about temporarily by a fever or after taking psychedelic drugs, but if they become chronic, they are cornerstone symptoms of a psychotic disorder. Here is a description of one person's experience of schizophrenia, written by the writer and former political aide Alastair Campbell about his brother Donald (emphasis in the original):

> The workings of your mind become separated from the reality around you. And it can be terrifying. Imagine a cacophony of voices in your head, screaming, telling you to do things you **normally** know you shouldn't. Then imagine plugs, sockets and light switches, road signs and shop signs talking to you. Imagine sitting in a place like this with a crowd like this and thinking every single word being said **and thought** by everyone is about **you**. Imagine watching TV and everyone is talking about you. And then imagine snakes coming out of the floor and wild cats charging through the walls and ceilings. Donald had all that and more when he was in a crisis.[1]

'Schizophrenia' is also a poorly understood term and is often used to refer to someone with a 'split personality', like

Dr Jekyll and Mr Hyde, but that's not what it means at all. It is possible for someone to display several apparently different personalities in this way, but this is instead referred to as dissociative identity disorder. In fact, schizophrenia involves psychotic symptoms combined with other symptoms such as difficulty processing and organising thoughts, and anhedonia (a loss of pleasure). Besides revealing how scary it must be to experience a psychotic episode like this, the above passage may make it hard to believe that delusions and hallucinations exist on a continuum. Surely you either believe or feel bizarre untrue things – like that the plug socket is talking to you – or you don't?

In fact, these symptoms exist on continua just like everything else. Take the example of auditory verbal hallucinations. These inner voices may appear to come from one or many people, and are typically negative, often saying distressing and frightening things. But auditory verbal hallucinations can vary in loudness and frequency; the content of them can vary; and people's relationship with them can differ: some people can exert more control over the voices than other people can, for example. A surprising proportion of 'healthy' people hear someone else talking inside their head – around 13% of adults in the general population.[2] These voice-hearers are *not* considered to have a mental illness because the voices they hear are less frequent, less negative, and/or easier to control. In other words, these people are on the lower end of a continuum of auditory verbal hallucinations.

As for delusions: think about how many people hold strong beliefs without any evidence, who believe in ghosts or UFOs, or that vaccinations cause autism, or that homeopathy has any effect beyond being a placebo, even when confronted with evidence to the contrary. Think about how many of us are superstitious – the person who wears the same 'lucky' T-shirt whenever they run a race, or touches wood to avoid something bad happening – or about the person who becomes fixated, just on a hunch, that their partner is cheating on them, or the person with the awful singing voice who goes on a TV talent show because they're convinced they're going to be a star.

'Beliefs in unscientific or parapsychological phenomena are not statistically uncommon ... and were this criterion alone employed as a sufficient condition, then many of us at times might be classified as delusional.' This was written by psychologists Vaughan Bell, Peter Halligan and Hadyn Ellis in 2003 in an article debating how to define delusions.[3] Religious beliefs also present a quandary, they said: they make the point that praying to a deity is not considered to be a delusion, whereas saying that one *is* a deity would be considered a delusion. In this respect, the culture and time in which someone lives are relevant in determining whether a belief is pathological. Paranormal or unscientific beliefs are only considered delusions if they aren't widely sanctioned by the person's culture or society.

Delusions might on the face of it seem like an obvious psychiatric symptom, but the line between them and 'normal', healthy beliefs is blurred. The point at which a belief usefully becomes a delusion is subtle, a matter of degree. As Bell and colleagues say, the decision about whether an individual is experiencing a delusion is often made 'on pragmatic grounds ... the extent of personal distress, potential or actual injury [to them or someone else] or social danger generated by the belief'. As a belief becomes more extreme on any of these factors, it might become useful to call it a delusion, but the distinction is not black and white. Delusions, in other words, are on a continuum.

Paranoia – a sense that others are talking about you or out to harm you – is one of the most common themes of delusions. As one group of researchers, led by psychologist Daniel Freeman, said: 'For many people, thoughts that friends, acquaintances or strangers might be hostile, or deliberately watching them, appear to be an everyday occurrence.'[4] One 2017 study led by Anam Elahi assessed the relationship between this kind of everyday paranoia and full-blown paranoid delusions like 'The neighbours are poisoning my water supply'.[5] The researchers used a questionnaire which asked over 2,800 respondents how much they agreed with statements such as 'There are times when I worry others might be plotting against me'. Some of the participants were randomly selected from the general population, some were known to be at risk of psychotic disorders (e.g. a member of their family had such a disorder), and some had a diagnosis of a psychotic disorder such as schizophrenia. When the researchers analysed all the data together, they found that it wasn't possible to draw a clear line between a delusional group and a non-delusional group; it was just one big, gradually changing group, with no sudden shift, no cliff edge, just a gradually smaller number of people experiencing an increasing severity of paranoia.

Here an important distinction made by Bell and colleagues comes into play: clinicians assessing a person will not only take into account whether the severity of the symptom crosses a certain numerical threshold, but will also make a clinical judgement of the *distress and disruption caused by that symptom* – and thus a pragmatic decision that the potential benefits of diagnosis and treatment outweigh any potential risks or downsides of such interventions. This is why those big epidemiological studies that rely on questionnaires alone, or clinical interviews carried out by non-experts, can pose a problem: this fine-tuned assessment of how much symptoms are actually affecting a person is critical in deciding whether any diagnosis or treatment is needed.

It is worth bearing in mind that this slippery, line-drawing business and this pragmatic exercising of clinical judgement is not just a problem for psychiatry; it's typical of many branches of medicine. Symptoms of many physical health conditions also exist on continua with no definitive point at which they become an illness or a disease. There is, for example, a continuum of renal function throughout the population: some people's kidneys work extremely well, others' slightly less so, others' only moderately well, and so on. The threshold at which suboptimal kidney function becomes chronic kidney disease does not exist in nature. The same is true of osteoarthritis, hypertension, obesity, gout, chronic obstructive pulmonary disease and many more. Just as in psychiatry, the threshold has to be artificially created, determined by experts.

At what point does anxiety become a disorder?

The continua we have discussed so far – low mood, auditory hallucinations and delusions – are all single symptoms, not disorders in themselves. As I said above, no diagnosis for a mental disorder is made based on one symptom alone. To illustrate how in practice the cut-off point for a full disorder is determined, a useful example is that of anxiety disorders, because pretty much everyone experiences some level of anxiety. So, how does clinical anxiety differ from the common anxiety that everyone experiences?

The *Diagnostic Statistical Manual of Mental Disorders* (DSM – the latest edition is known as DSM-5) compiled by the American Psychiatric Association is often referred to as the 'bible' of psychiatric disorders.[6] It's not the only such categorisation system – there's the *International Classification of Diseases* (ICD-11), for example, published by the World Health Organisation, which groups and defines mental disorders in a slightly different way. As will become apparent over the course of this book, the DSM – and the idea of categorising mental disorders at all – has been criticised. But it is a useful starting point for understanding how mental illness is currently classified.

Anxiety takes two forms, panic and worry. In most DSM anxiety disorders, both processes can become dysfunctional, although the relative emphasis on each can vary. Panic is the physical side of anxiety, the physiological way that your body reacts when you're afraid. It's the way you might feel when you're walking somewhere deserted at night, or when someone threatens you, or when you're flying and the plane goes through a bad patch of turbulence: light-headedness, racing heart, sweaty palms. The other component of anxiety, worry, resides in the mind. Worry – its official name, even in the academic literature – is the cognitive process of thinking negative thoughts, typically about the future; it's the process of holding on to these thoughts, going over and over them. You might worry about minor things like missing your train or about how your social media post will be received, or bigger, more serious things like how your cancer will affect your family, or about losing your job or your housing. Worries essentially revolve around bad things happening, disaster striking.

So far, so familiar. Feeling fear in your body and having worries in your mind are entirely normal experiences, part and parcel of being alive. In fact, as every therapist loves to tell you in session one: we need *some* level of anxiety, both panic and worry. An entire absence of anxiety would get us into all kinds of trouble. But anxiety disorders occur when these common processes get completely out of control.

When panic reaches its extreme state, it becomes a panic attack. Like many terms relating to mental illness, this phrase has a colloquial meaning that bears very little relation to the clinical one. At the time of writing, someone recently tweeted that they had a panic attack looking at James Corden in the trailer for the new film *Cats*. I've watched the trailer and it's not a pretty sight, granted, but I'd bet good money that this person didn't actually have a panic attack. In everyday parlance, 'panic attack' has become shorthand for being suddenly stressed or shocked. The reality of panic attacks is quite different and specific. In a panic attack, a person becomes so overwhelmed with the physical experience of anxiety that they start to feel that they can't breathe, which then sets off a horrible spiral: as they take too many quick, short breaths, they begin to hyperventilate. The resulting increased exhalation decreases the amount of carbon dioxide in their blood, causing more symptoms of panic – like dizziness, nausea and chest pains. During a panic attack, people often feel like they are going into cardiac arrest or dying, and sometimes call the emergency services. Panic attacks can last up to twenty minutes: an agonisingly long period to be in such an intense state of fear. They can be triggered in the face of sudden danger or overwhelmingly stressful life circumstances, or they can be triggered by very little.

A panic attack alone is not a mental illness. There is a disorder in the DSM which is primarily defined by panic attacks, panic disorder, but two criteria must be met: the panic attacks must be recurrent, and one of them must have been followed by at least a month of worry about the attacks – the person fears they will have another attack, and starts to change their behaviour (e.g. not going to certain places) in order to reduce their risk. Sadly, just as panic attacks themselves are vicious cycles, the experience of having a panic attack can set up an intense fear of having another one, which in itself can trigger the very event that is feared. Only once a person is in this cycle – a persistent pattern of attacks and fear about attacks – would a professional consider a diagnosis of panic *disorder*. Interestingly, the initial source of the panic, if one can be found, is not part of the equation in the DSM. In theory, people could be diagnosed with this disorder even if the panic seems to be quite a logical response to an incredibly stressful situation.

The thinking side of anxiety is worry. Psychologists often point out that worry and rumination (common in depression) are both patterns of repetitive negative thinking – which is one reason why anxiety and depression so often occur together – but that worries are more about the future while ruminative thoughts tend to be about the past. We are all probably familiar with the idea that some people tend to worry more often than others, irrespective of what is going on in their lives, envisaging things going wrong frequently and devising all kinds of potential problems in their head. People who do this a lot are often dismissed as just 'worriers'. But at what point does a worrier become someone who has an anxiety disorder?

There are a number of different factors that academics and clinicians – including the people writing the DSM – look at when it comes to working out whether worry (or any other mental health problem) has reached pathological levels, some of which have already been mentioned. The first is *chronicity*: how long has this person been worrying a lot? A week or months? Is the worry there most days, or just occasionally? The second is *severity:* have the worries been mild or difficult or overwhelming? The third is *disruption*, as discussed before: has the worry stopped the person being able to function normally in their daily life? And related to all of this is *control*: is the person able to manage their worries and reason their way out of them or not? All of these factors are taken into account to determine whether someone is a bit of a worrier, compared to someone who might usefully be considered to have a disorder.

People with generalised anxiety disorder (GAD) have a pathological problem with worry: they experience a frequent stream of exaggerated concerns about various different scenarios. There are lots of other anxiety disorders; what distinguishes GAD is its focus on worry (rather than panic) and the fact that the content of the worries is broad, hence 'generalised'. It was GAD that I was diagnosed with, along with depression, back when I was twenty. I've heard GAD described as 'worrying about anything and everything', although I've never identified with this description. In fact, part of the reason I'm reluctant to admit I was diagnosed with GAD is that I don't want people to assume I worry about everything. I don't, and even at my worst I never did. It's just that the content of the worry in GAD is *relatively* broad, compared to say, social anxiety disorder or a phobia of snakes.

In the current DSM, in order to meet criteria for GAD, you need to tick each of the following boxes. First, you need to have worried 'excessively' for more days than not each week, for at least six months, and about many different things. Second, you must find it difficult to control the worry, and third, you must be showing at least three of the following physical symptoms over the same time period: feeling restless or on edge; being easily fatigued; having difficulty concentrating; irritability; muscle tension or sleep disturbance.

By the time I was diagnosed with GAD, I had had an obsessive problem with worry not just for six months, but more like ten years. I have a distinct memory of the first time I had a GAD-type worry, actually: I was nine or ten, in a geography class at school, looking at a huge world map that spanned the wall behind my teacher. Like a lightning bolt, a thought appeared in my head, crystal clear: my mum had been killed in a car crash, and she would never come and pick me up from school. By the time the school day finished – and she appeared, no problem – I was a mess. I'm sure I was anxious before then, but in my memory that moment marks the start, the beginning of many years of frequent, excessive anxious thoughts. From then on, my mind was riddled with private, absurd worries that I couldn't control.

For me, GAD sometimes felt like a vague, all-encompassing sense of dread – like when you're watching a film and you hear suspenseful music playing, and you know for certain that something awful is about to happen, you just don't know what. At other times, pathological worries arrived suddenly, fully formed. These were detailed and specific – the people involved, the precise sequence of events: a razor-sharp nightmare played out in the theatre of my mind before I'd even had time to blink. Even though much therapy has taught me that the vividness of these scenarios bears no relation to their likelihood of happening, this can be difficult to accept. When they occasionally still appear, the images feel as real and true as a punch in the face.

In my childhood and teenage years, I kept the extent of my anxiety to myself. My parents knew I worried, and that there were certain things I was extremely reluctant to do because of it, but they had no idea how bad it was. This was partly because I didn't tell them, but it was also because they had no framework or context to realise that worry *could* be that bad, because no one talked about this stuff back then. And there's no way I would ever have told my friends, wouldn't have even contemplated it. The worries were a constant part of my existence, but an entirely silent and private one. I don't know if I was ashamed about them, as such. I just didn't talk about it. No one did.

I was never aware that I might have a disorder. Up until university I thought worrying was just part of who I was – a tiresome, exhausting corner of my identity – and even doing a psychology degree wasn't enough to make me realise that I might have a treatable problem. In fact, I remember reading about GAD as a first-year undergraduate and thinking: boy, that sounds bad. Even with the description right in front of me, I didn't make the link with my own experience, not until things got considerably worse.

The crucial thing to notice – from my own experience and the professional approach – is that 'normal' worry and the pathological worry seen in GAD are distinguished on multiple different criteria: the severity of the symptoms, the frequency, the chronicity, the controllability, and the extent to which they impact on daily functioning. The cut-offs in each of these criteria are pretty arbitrary – someone who otherwise met all GAD criteria but who had worried excessively only for five months rather than six, for example, would still have a serious issue with worry. Indeed, not quite reaching this boundary doesn't mean you'll be turned away from treatment. As I've said, mental health professionals are rarely wedded to precise DSM criteria – they are usually more concerned with the impact that symptoms are having on a person's life, and they exercise their judgement about the value and necessity of a diagnosis and intervention. But by dividing each disorder into a suite of symptoms and assessing each symptom on the basis of several criteria, clinicians and researchers can at least have an approximate shared understanding of what constitutes a disorder – despite the fact that the symptoms of mental illness will always lie on a smooth continuum with normal human experience, and the line delineating where mental illness begins will always be imperfect.

Having found a way to manage this problem, however, we soon meet another. The multiplicity of symptoms that make up each disorder mean that, for some disorders, two people with the same diagnosis might actually have quite a different set of problems.

The many variations of depression

If you've known more than one person with depression, or if you've experienced it yourself and also seen someone else go through it, you'll have noticed that individual experiences of depression can be very different. Some have difficulty getting out of bed because they are sleeping so much, while others can't sleep at all. Some seem slow and lethargic while others seem to have a lot of irritable, agitated energy. How can these different symptoms usefully form the basis of the same diagnosis?

For a long time, it's been recognised that depression is about much more than low mood. This isn't to dismiss this part of the disorder; the low mood alone is dark and desperate. William Styron, in his highly influential memoir *Darkness Visible*, wrote that depressed mood is 'so mysteriously painful and elusive … as to verge close to being beyond description. It thus remains nearly incomprehensible to those who have not experienced it in its extreme mode.'[7] But the low mood combines with many other symptoms. For those charged with diagnosing the disorder, according to DSM-5, there are nine possible symptoms to consider:

1. Depressed mood most of the day, nearly every day.
2. Markedly diminished interest or pleasure in all, or almost all, activities most of the day, nearly every day.
3. Significant weight loss when not dieting or weight gain, or decrease or increase in appetite nearly every day.

4. Insomnia (inability to get to sleep or difficulty staying asleep) or hypersomnia (sleeping too much) nearly every day.
5. A slowing down of thought and a reduction of physical movement (observable by others, not merely subjective feelings of restlessness or being slowed down).
6. Fatigue or loss of energy nearly every day.
7. Feelings of worthlessness or excessive or inappropriate guilt nearly every day.
8. Diminished ability to think or concentrate, or indecisiveness, nearly every day.
9. Recurrent thoughts of death, recurrent suicidal ideation without a specific plan, or a suicide attempt or a specific plan for suicide.

The reason that we encounter so many different versions of depression is because a person need only experience five out of these nine symptoms to meet the official criteria. (Each symptom needs to have been there most of the time for at least two weeks, and must be affecting the person's ability to function in their daily life.) At least one of the five must be either low mood or loss of pleasure from things you used to enjoy. This is known as anhedonia (mentioned previously as being also a symptom of schizophrenia) and is perfectly captured by the journalist Mark Rice-Oxley when describing how he felt about tinkering on the piano – which he had once loved – when he was depressed: 'Now when I sit at the piano, none of this seems relevant or captivating. I just stare at the keys. I cannot think what could possibly have made it interesting to play the piano. I cannot think what could possibly have been interesting about listening to music. I can't hear it anymore. It's all just noise.'[8]

Thus, according to the DSM-5 guidelines, it's actually possible to have depression and not even be experiencing low mood at all – although one study found that low mood was the most common depression symptom, reported by almost 94%

of patients.⁹ All in all, there are a full 227 different possible combinations of these symptoms that could get you a diagnosis of depression. On top of this, because some of the symptoms have a few different options (e.g. feelings of worthlessness *or* guilt), it's possible to have two people with depression who have no overlapping symptoms at all, and because some of the symptoms include their opposite – you might be sleeping too much *or* not enough (number 4); or have experienced an increase *or* decrease in weight (3) – two people with depression can be experiencing some entirely opposing symptoms.

The search for subtypes

This suggests that depression is not really one single disorder. Instead, depression may be better thought of as an umbrella term for a host of different disorders – in the same way that the term 'cancer' incorporates disorders such as leukaemia, sarcoma and breast cancer that are distinct from one another. But even though most experts know that there *are* different versions of depression, no one can tie down exactly what those subtypes are. Having clearly specified sub-disorders would be useful, because each subtype may have different causes and, importantly, different treatments. If we could diagnose specific types of depression, more targeted treatments could be offered, reducing suffering and improving outcomes. But unlike with cancer, researchers have not been able to clearly figure out what these different types of depression might be. At the moment, treating depression takes a trial-and-error approach, in which a series of different medications and therapies are prescribed one after the other, in the hope that one is found to be effective.

This imprecision is not for lack of trying. Researchers have attempted to make distinctions between different types of depression based on various features: associated symptoms (e.g. anxious depression, psychotic depression), causes (e.g. depression that starts in pregnancy, depression that occurs after a life event), or the age at which it starts (adolescent versus adult onset).[10] But every attempt to find consistent categories has been thwarted, either because too many people fall into more than one category (for example, a person who is depressed in pregnancy could also have had prior depressive episodes with different triggers), and/or because too many people don't fall into any group at all. It may be that there are just too many different ways to be depressed – each one so tied up in the unique and complex circumstances of the sufferer – that it's impossible to have a constrained list of depression subtypes. Or we may just not have worked it out yet: the science of mental illness is young, and things are changing all the time. For now, all we have is one label, depression, its breadth reminding us once again that catching and fencing off mental illness is a rather tricky thing to do.

The writer Esmé Weijun Wang, whose mood problems and psychosis were first diagnosed as bipolar disorder and later as schizoaffective disorder, summed up her thoughts on the DSM-5 (which is a deep purple colour): 'It is easy to forget that psychiatric diagnoses are human constructs, and not handed down from an all-knowing God on stone tablets; to "have schizophrenia" is to fit an assemblage of symptoms, which are listed in a purple book made by humans.'[11]

This idea of psychiatric diagnoses being human constructs is an important one that we will return to throughout this book. And I'm afraid to say that it doesn't get any simpler from here. Not only is it difficult to draw the line between mental health and illness, or the lines around different illnesses: the official position of where the lines ought to be drawn keeps on changing, every few years. This is the topic we turn to next.

CHAPTER 3

Moving goalposts

If I asked you to guess how many different disorders appear in the DSM-5, what would you say? We've mentioned a few so far, like depression and OCD, and you have likely heard of some others, like anorexia. It would be reasonable to assume that the total number is quite high, given the sheer vastness of human experience. Consider every facet of your life: every day is made up of thousands of different thoughts, emotions, decisions, actions; throughout your life you experience countless aspects of being human. Any one of these can go wrong. There are disorders relating to sleep, sex and substance use; there are disorders of attention, impulse control and personality. There is a pathological version of every other human thought process, emotion and behaviour you can imagine too: a version where it becomes so extreme (or so entirely absent) that it impacts on a person's ability to function.

When the first edition of the DSM was published in 1952, it listed 106 disorders, and with each subsequent iteration, that number has grown. In fact that number has now grown so much that researchers cannot agree on how many different diagnostic categories actually appear in the DSM-5. This is because it depends what you count as a distinct disorder – is gambling disorder (episodic) distinct from gambling disorder (persistent) for these purposes? And what about stimulant use disorder where the drug is amphetamine versus stimulant use disorder involving cocaine? In both these examples, the clinician is asked to 'specify' which category the patient falls into, but it's up for debate how distinct they actually are. When describing the total number of diagnoses in the DSM-5, some researchers give the more cautious figure of 298,[1] others simply say 'over 400',[2] others say it is as high as 541.[3] Whatever the exact figure, there is wide agreement that each time the DSM is updated, the number gets bigger. The first edition had 128 pages; DSM-5 has 947.

One possible reason for this is that over time we have discovered the existence of more disorders. But when DSM-5 was published in 2013, there was a cascade of criticism of it, which raised a second possibility. Maybe we're now labelling too many psychological experiences as disorders, applying the term 'mental illness' to things that shouldn't be called illnesses at all. Because in almost all cases, the boundaries around what is officially considered to be an illness are expanding.

Across each iteration of the DSM, the list of disorders has expanded in two ways. Nicholas Haslam, a psychologist from Australia, refers to this as vertical and horizontal expansion.[4] Vertical expansion is when the threshold for an existing disorder is lowered: the severity with which something must be experienced to reach a diagnosis has been reduced. Horizontal expansion refers to the fact that, in Haslam's words, 'an increasingly wide assortment of psychological phenomena [now] fall within the psychiatric domain'.[5] Existing disorders are being extended to include more symptoms, and entirely new disorders are being described. The upshot is that more and more types of human experience are being labelled as problematic – a phenomenon he refers to as 'concept creep'.

The history of social anxiety disorder

Social anxiety disorder (SAD) is a case in point that usefully illustrates what is happening. SAD is an anxiety disorder characterised by intense, persistent worry or panic related to situations with other people, particularly those in which the individual will be judged or evaluated in some way. People with SAD are not just shy: fear about these situations is so intense that it becomes utterly debilitating. They might worry about social situations weeks in advance, or avoid them altogether, and experience panic attacks when in social situations or when contemplating them. One teenage participant, in a Norwegian study about the impact of social anxiety, described it like this:

> Everything becomes difficult, you get so insanely aware of how extremely social even the smallest things are. You have to meet people's gazes ... and you sort of have to be a part of a large society. When I'm having a good day then I do not think about how many people I actually meet, or how many people I have to interact with. But when the bad days come, then I have to prepare myself for everything really, think a lot about the smallest details and feel that it's hard to do things.[6]

Another participant in a study conducted in Iran said simply, 'Social anxiety has ruined my life. I am always worried about social situations.'[7]

In the DSM-5, a person must meet the following criteria to reach a diagnosis of SAD. The feared social situations almost always provoke anxiety, the anxiety is out of proportion to the threat, the person starts to avoid the situations (or endures them with intense anxiety), and the anxiety causes significant distress. All of this must be persistent, typically lasting for at least six months. (Note again how a person must be experiencing an *intense* and *debilitating* amount of social anxiety to have social anxiety *disorder*; many people experience milder levels of social anxiety, which in the past would probably just have been called shyness.)

In 1980 (DSM-III), however, social anxiety disorder (then called social phobia) was exclusively about fear of performance scenarios, like public speaking. In 1994 (DSM-IV), the name was changed to social anxiety disorder, and the subject of the fear was broadened to include any social situations in which a person is exposed to 'unfamiliar people or possible scrutiny by others'. This is an example of horizontal expansion. Being evaluated is an obvious consequence of scenarios like public speaking, but most social interactions involve some element of being judged, and people who are prone to social anxiety can be intensely worried about a whole range of social situations that aren't about public performance: eating in public, phoning someone they don't know well or entering a room when others are already seated, for example. Obviously there were people before 1994 who felt anxious about these scenarios, and I've no doubt that for some of them, the anxiety was so debilitating it caused untold distress and difficulty in their lives. It's just that, rightly or wrongly, they wouldn't have been considered to have a mental illness. Back then, you were diagnosed as having SAD only if your anxiety was about performing in public.

The definition of SAD has also expanded vertically in the DSM-5. In the previous iteration of the manual, there was a specification that in individuals under eighteen years old, the anxiety needed to be present for at least six months. In the most recent edition, a diagnosis is warranted for people of all ages if the anxiety is 'persistent, typically lasting six months or more'. This fairly small change in wording means that a young person who had experienced social anxiety for four months, say, could now meet the official diagnostic criteria for SAD.

There are plenty of other examples. Bulimia is defined by a pattern of uncontrollable binging (enormously excessive eating, often tens of thousands of calories at a time, often to the point – intentionally – of being in physical pain) and purging (behaviours to counteract weight gain, like self-induced vomiting, extreme exercise or taking laxatives). But doctors and researchers noticed that some people frequently binge-eat, and have immense difficulty controlling this behaviour, but do not purge. Clearly these individuals have a dysfunctional relationship with food. So the new diagnostic label of binge-eating disorder, which doesn't require purging, was created.

A similar expansion happened with bipolar disorder, a type of mood disorder in which people cycle through episodes of depression and mania (hence its former name, manic depression). Mania is a period of elated mood and associated symptoms, such as sudden increases in self-esteem, increased energy and reduced need for sleep. These might sound like good things but episodes of mania are deeply unpleasant and frightening: one's mood can be so elevated that you feel wired and irritable, experiencing racing thoughts or speech. The erratic burst of energy and confidence leads people to do things like spend money they don't have, get into fights or cheat on their partner. The writer Hattie Gladwell spent £3,000 on tattoos during a period of mania:

> That's what I felt when I went into the tattoo shop. Adrenaline. The type you'd get when you reached the top of a super-high roller coaster, ready to go down to the bottom. I'd already had three tattoos – but over the course of two months, I was covered in twenty-six. I covered my legs, my stomach, my back, my neck and my arms … It started when I made friends with a girl who was also covered in tattoos – I'd always thought she looked amazing but wasn't sure if I could go through with that myself, dedicating a lifetime to ink on my body. I'd considered it, and there were times where I was tempted to head to the tattoo studio, but I always chickened out, thinking more rationally: would I regret this? But when I was manic, I didn't think about those things.[8]

At some point, psychologists noticed that some individuals had problematic episodes of elevated mood and unpredictable behaviour similar to but less extreme than this. The term 'hypomania' was therefore introduced – a slightly milder version of mania – and ultimately a new version of bipolar disorder was created, 'bipolar disorder II', to describe the experience of episodes of depression paired with episodes of the slightly milder hypomania.

But as the DSM has swelled to include more variants of psychological experience – more symptoms, or less extreme versions of symptoms – perhaps the most significant expansion has been with a deceptively simple term: trauma.

At what point does response to a traumatic event become a mental illness?

On 7 July 2005, I was in the sixth-form common room at my school when someone received a text from their dad, who worked in London. He said there had been a terrorist attack. I remember lots of other students then texting and calling their own parents, as many of them commuted to London for work. This was before the days of social media or Internet on mobile phones, so it took a while for the details to emerge. But within a few days, we had the facts. Four terrorists had detonated bombs on three Tube trains and one bus during the morning rush hour. Fifty-two people were killed, more than 700 were injured: still the deadliest terrorist attack to have happened in the UK. Ten years later, my PhD office was just across the road from Tavistock Square, where the final bomb went off on a bus. On the ten-year anniversary, there was a short service in Tavistock Square Gardens, and the classical music that was played, which drifted into our office that morning, was heartbreaking.

Unsurprisingly, many of the survivors of this attack suffered long-term psychological effects, and some of them were subsequently diagnosed with post-traumatic stress disorder. PTSD is characterised by repeated intrusive memories of an event, like nightmares or flashbacks; a tendency to avoid triggers of the memories; and negative emotions like depression or irritability. People with this disorder become locked into a harrowing re-experiencing of what happened to them, feeling the horror of the event in their mind and body again and again, to the point where they can scarcely engage with their current life. If they do not receive the right help, people with PTSD can suffer for decades.

The key thing about PTSD that sets it apart from other diagnoses is that there is a specific triggering event: the trauma. In recent years, the term PTSD has become more commonplace, partly because the definition of the word 'trauma' has been getting wider. Originally, the word was used to refer to a physical injury, as in 'blunt force trauma'. In psychiatry, therefore, it referred to a physical injury to the brain. It is still used in that way, as in the term 'traumatic brain injury'. However, in 1980 (DSM-III) the disorder PTSD first appeared, and there the word was used to refer to an event that causes severe psychological harm (often accompanying physical injury). In order to be considered traumatic, the triggering event had to meet several strict criteria. It had to be so extreme that it would evoke significant distress in almost anyone, it had to be outside what is normally experienced, and it had to present a real or imagined threat to the person's life. So being in a serious accident, natural disaster or violent crime would have counted. As would, of course, a terrorist attack. So far, so reasonable. No one would dispute that experiencing these awful events has the capacity to cause serious psychological harm.

But there was a problem: some people develop symptoms of PTSD even when their own life isn't at risk but when they witness *someone else's* life at risk – this can happen in first responders like paramedics and police officers. In the 2005 London terrorist attack, the London Ambulance Service deployed fifty vehicles and more than 250 staff to help the injured. Two months after the bombings, psychologists conducted a study to assess symptoms of PTSD in those who helped.[9] They found that 4% of the sample had sufficiently severe symptoms that they met criteria for PTSD (note it was all done by questionnaire, and a definitive diagnosis should be given by a trained clinician). A further 13% exhibited substantial distress (reporting at least one of ten possible PTSD symptoms, like 'being jumpy at something unexpected' or 'upsetting dreams about the event'). According to the original definition of trauma, people like this wouldn't have met criteria for PTSD, because their own life wasn't at risk, so the criteria were expanded to include people who had witnessed others' lives at risk, not just their own.

This seems to me a perfectly reasonable adjustment: it must be harrowing to attend some of these scenes, which is why I admire, so much, all the first responders that do. But what if the definition included not only those who witnessed another's life at risk but also those who learn at a distance of a loved-one's life being at risk? In the latest edition of the DSM, trauma now also includes *indirect* exposure: 'learning about violent or accidental death, serious harm or threat of death or injury experienced by a family member or other close associate'. For example, a person might develop PTSD in the aftermath of their child being in an accident, even though they weren't there, or after their partner was seriously injured in a violent assault. Again, this isn't unreasonable: learning about these events, and dealing with their aftermath, could be horrifying.

And then: what if you didn't witness the event, and it didn't happen to someone you love – could hearing about frightening events happening to strangers trigger PTSD? In the DSM-5 it was decided that you *could* develop PTSD in this indirect way, but only if it was part of your job – for example, as a 999 operator answering calls about a terrorist attack, a psychotherapist supporting a torture victim, or a police officer reviewing evidence of child abuse. The next time a diagnostic manual is published, the definition will likely have changed again. As clinical psychologist Vaughan Bell says: 'The fact that we have these increasingly convoluted definitions shows that we are still trying to negotiate the borders of what is considered to be traumatic.'[10]

Trauma is hard to define because, as US psychologists Frank Weathers and Terence Keane explain, 'there are no crisp boundaries demarcating ordinary stressors from traumatic stressors'.[11] This is the problem we have already come up against with symptoms of mental illness. But trauma is also hard to define because not everyone who lives through highly stressful events develops PTSD – in fact, the majority don't (more on that later).

Which raises a tricky question: if someone survives a violent assault, say, and doesn't develop symptoms of PTSD, was the assault a trauma? Equally: if someone experiences something fairly commonplace and *does* develop such symptoms, does the event become a trauma by default? If we take the view that a person's response to an event, rather than the event itself, should determine what 'counts' as a trauma, then potentially anything could. The upshot of grappling with these questions, and the resultant horizontal expansion, is that responses to an increasingly wide range of distressing life experiences now have the potential to be categorised as traumas – and the response to them mental disorders.

Finding trauma everywhere

Not only do we see PTSD where we didn't see it before, we actively look for it in places we wouldn't previously have thought to. In one study, 769 university students were asked how they felt about the 2016 election of President Trump, two or three months after the event.[12] Another recent study collected data from seventy-three students who had been cheated on by a long-term romantic partner in the last five years.[13] Both studies considered their respective events (Trump's election, a partner's infidelity) to be a potential trauma, and wanted to screen for resulting symptoms of PTSD in their samples.

In both studies, participants were given a questionnaire called the Impact of Events Scale, which is a measure of twenty-two PTSD symptoms. Example items include 'I had dreams about (the event)' and 'Reminders of (the event) have caused me to have physical reactions such as sweating, trouble breathing, nausea or a pounding heart'. Respondents report how much each statement reflects their experience, from 1 (Not at all) to 4 (Often true). Of a maximum score of 88, previous researchers have suggested that 33 or above indicates 'probable PTSD', and this cut-off was adopted in both these studies. On that basis, the researchers found that 25% of the students in the

Trump study and 45% of those in the infidelity study met this threshold.

It is important to note that neither study goes so far as to say these people actually have PTSD – that would require evaluation by a clinician. But that distinction gets lost when studies such as these are reported in mainstream media: 'College kids blame Trump for PTSD' read the *New York Post*'s headline, for example. This is how an agony aunt in *The Atlantic* recently answered a letter from a man whose partner had been unfaithful:

> First, you should know that your reaction is completely understandable in the aftermath of infidelity. In fact, what you're describing is a common response to trauma. I use the word trauma because while most people can easily imagine (or are personally acquainted with) the pain of being cheated on, what some may not realize is that many betrayed partners experience symptoms of PTSD.[14]

This may be so, but merely thinking a lot about an event is a symptom of PTSD. It doesn't mean you *have* PTSD, just as experiencing a low mood (a symptom of depression) doesn't mean you are depressed. Symptoms only become a disorder if you experience a lot of them, at an intense level, for a long time. Otherwise they are just negative emotions, thoughts and behaviours: normal, albeit unpleasant, human experiences. But now, in the media and public discussion (a subject we will return to later), this nuance is getting lost. Individual and relatively mild symptoms of a mental illness are frequently conflated with the disorder itself.

Trump's election was devastating for numerous Americans, particularly many people of colour, Muslims, immigrants, LGBT+ people, and those fighting for women's rights, progressive ideals and the environment, according to one paper by academic Beth Sondel and colleagues.[15] Likewise, discovering a partner's infidelity can be profoundly distressing: it can entirely upend your life, changing your understanding of yourself, your relationship, your past and your future. But if we call all stressful events traumas – originally only used to describe events like war and torture and terrorist attacks – and call all resulting distress PTSD, what words are left for the people who lose a limb in a terrorist attack, say? Later in this book, we'll look at how this expansion of mental health terms like PTSD can erode their value for everyone.

Are there upsides to expansion?

In the DSM-IV, there was an important note in the section about major depressive disorder. It instructed clinicians not to diagnose depression if the person – who seems to be presenting with symptoms of depression – has recently suffered a bereavement. The rationale was that when someone you love has just died, the distress that you display is grief, a *normal* response to loss. For the more recent DSM-5, this 'bereavement exclusion' was removed – one of the manual's most controversial revisions. It now says that as long as someone has been experiencing symptoms for two weeks (a widely agreed minimum time frame for depressive symptoms), they can be diagnosed with depression, *even if those two weeks followed the death of a loved one.* This means that if your partner dies suddenly and fifteen days later you are still experiencing symptoms like crying frequently and having difficulty sleeping, you could be told you are experiencing a mental illness, diagnosed with major depression and prescribed antidepressants.

The decision to remove the bereavement exclusion remains a contentious one, and a number of researchers and psychiatrists have written in protest about it, saying that this is turning grief into a mental illness – academics Chris Dowrick and Allen Frances described it as a 'medical intrusion into private emotions'.[16] But this adjustment was not made without a great deal of thought. The researchers and clinicians who made this decision rationalised it like this: just because a loved one has recently died, doesn't mean you can't *also* be hit by depression.

They argue that depression is clearly distinguishable from typical grief: for example, depression is unrelenting, whereas the emotions of grief typically come in waves.[17] People experiencing typical grief are more able to experience positive emotions, to have hope for the future, and to have a positive view of themselves – all of which differs from people with depression. So if someone is hit by both bereavement and depression, the idea goes, we should attempt to treat and support the depression, just as we would for someone who hadn't suffered a loss. As we conduct more research and develop more understanding, it's perhaps no bad thing that we continue to refine and redefine our guidelines in this way.

Other aspects of concept creep in recent decades have clearly been right and helpful. In the earliest editions of the DSM, for example, there was very limited recognition that children or adolescents could have mental illness. There was a single, vaguely defined category called 'adjustment reaction of childhood/adolescence', which referred to difficulty coping with life events, but that was it. Now, there is extensive evidence that it's not only possible to develop mental illness before adulthood, but that actually this is when the majority of cases begin (which we discuss further in Chapter 6). It was right that this expansion was made.

Like the grief example, expanding boundaries can also make help available to more people who might need it. Binge-eating disorder and bipolar disorder II, for example, were added in recognition that some people show problematic symptoms that cause them significant distress and would benefit from help and treatment, but previously their lack of a diagnosis meant they had no access to treatment – particularly somewhere like the US, where a diagnosis is required for health insurance purposes. Similarly, expansion of the original definition of PTSD was sensible. If a police officer is having disabling flashbacks and panic attacks because of what she saw in the aftermath of a terrorist attack, she shouldn't be denied treatment just because her own life hadn't been at risk.

It's also worth noting that some disorders, such as sadistic personality disorder and Asperger's syndrome, have been removed from the DSM. (People who were previously diagnosed with Asperger's fall under autism spectrum disorder in the latest edition.) One particularly significant removal, of course, was that of homosexuality, which was listed as a mental disorder in the DSM until 1987. Even though overall the number of phenomena covered is increasing, the DSM is not blindly casting its net wider and wider. When appropriate, experiences that were once considered disorders have been either absorbed into other categories or dropped altogether. One 2020 meta-analysis by Fabian Fabiano and Nicholas Haslam found that while adjustments to *some* disorders in the DSM-5 have resulted in a higher potential rate of diagnoses, others have not – meaning that when you look across multiple disorders (they looked at forty-one), there is not much change since the previous edition in how many people meet criteria for 'a mental illness'.[18]

Nonetheless, there is considerable concern that vertical and horizontal expansion in some corners of the DSM – combined with public-awareness campaigns – will affect the way people understand their personalities or distress. Since the inception of the DSM in 1952, more people, accurately or not, will have some of their experiences labelled as psychological disorders, or be inclined to label them this way themselves. Psychiatrist Allen Frances, who chaired the task force who created the DSM-IV (1994), argues that the latest edition of the manual has contributed to this:

> The diagnostic exuberance of DSM-5 confuses mental disorder with the everyday sadness, anxiety, grief, disappointments, and stress responses that are an inescapable part of the human condition. DSM-5 ambitiously mislabels normal diversity and childhood immaturity as disorder, creating stigma and promoting the excess use of medications. We need a Goldilocks just-right balance between the risks of missing patients and of mislabeling them. At the moment, mislabeling rules.[19]

Might there only be one mental illness?

In parallel to all this expansion, a very different idea is being explored. Some researchers argue that instead of assuming each disorder is distinct, and dividing them into more and more refined categories, we should look at what they have in common. They argue we should focus on the broad underlying dysfunctions that are 'transdiagnostic' – common across disorders.

This idea has emerged for several reasons. First, lots of people with mental illness have more than one disorder. Most people (63%) who meet criteria for one disorder in their lifetime will meet criteria for a second one. Of those with two disorders, 53% will at some point meet criteria for a third; 41% with three will meet criteria for a fourth.[20] People often move from one disorder to another across time: they might have an anxiety disorder in childhood, then depression in their teen years, then schizophrenia in their early twenties, for example. If it's so common to slide between disorders, or have more than one of them at the same time, this suggests there might be something tying them all together.

The second fact is that, as we'll see over the next few chapters, different disorders often have similar causes. The same genes and stressful life events increase the risk of lots of different disorders. Third, a lot of symptoms, like anhedonia or delusions, appear in more than one disorder. (This has sometimes led to new diagnoses: some people show the mood extremes of bipolar disorder and the delusions and hallucinations of schizophrenia, leading to the hybrid diagnosis of 'schizoaffective disorder'.) Finally, the same treatments, like antidepressants or cognitive behavioural therapy, are effective for many different disorders. This all points to one possibility: perhaps different mental disorders aren't quite as distinct as we thought.

If many disorders derive from similar, or even the same, underlying dysfunctions, this would explain why symptoms cross diagnostic boundaries, why the same causes lead to different disorders, and why the same treatments help. The question worth investigating, then, is this: what are the core deficits or issues that are familiar across many different mental illnesses?

Psychologists Avshalom Caspi and Terrie Moffitt propose four possible dysfunctions.[21] The first is a general tendency toward negative emotional states and negative thoughts – the repetitive negative thinking like worry and rumination that I mentioned earlier. As we all know from our own pool of friends and family, some people are more susceptible than others to slipping into and staying in these negative states. This is captured by the personality trait neuroticism, which, like all personality traits, exists on a spectrum. Those at the high end are much more likely to develop disorders like anxiety disorders and depression – if the negative emotions and thoughts to which they are predisposed become overwhelming and dysfunctional. Relatedly, some people are also less able to regulate and dampen down those emotions once they appear. As we'll see, poor emotion regulation is relevant across many disorders.

A second common factor across many disorders is poor impulse control. This could mean saying or doing inappropriate things, especially when upset or angry; overreacting to certain experiences and events, including one's own thoughts; or impulsive behaviour like binge eating, excessive alcohol consumption, or gambling. Thirdly, poor executive function – the set of mental processes that allow us to maintain attention, work out problems and make decisions in a timely way – is common across many disorders. Finally, there is a transdiagnostic tendency to have unwanted irrational thoughts. These may at first glance seem to be exclusive to psychotic disorders like schizophrenia, but irrationality is fundamental to many psychiatric problems, including all the anxiety disorders. People with anorexia who are dangerously underweight believe they are fat; people with OCD often believe that they can control events (like a death in the family) by carrying out compulsions; many people with depression believe they are worthless and unlovable. (The concept of irrationality is somewhat controversial in mental illness – some researchers argue that thoughts that appear irrational on the face of it actually make some sense in the context of that person's history and circumstances – but it's still broadly true that many disorders involve holding extreme beliefs regardless of evidence to the contrary.)

If so many of these underlying tendencies are common to multiple disorders, the question then becomes: why do they manifest themselves in such a variety of ways? If two people have very poor impulse control, for example, why does one of them develop bulimia while the other one develops gambling disorder? (Of course, some people could wind up with both disorders.) We don't know the answer for sure yet. But it's possible that different disorders simply result from slightly different combinations of the same deficits and dysfunctions, in different quantities and ratios.

How these then combine with the different external context of each individual will also be important. For example, a person who tends to have intrusive and disordered thoughts who is then bullied at school may be more likely to develop psychosis or social anxiety disorder, while a similarly vulnerable person whose partner has just died may be more likely to develop depression or PTSD. A group of researchers led by psychologist Warren Mansell have described this as the person's 'current concerns' – whatever it is that is particularly salient or important in that person's life at that time will determine which specific disorder they end up having.[22] And what determines what specific concerns you will have? Well, a bit of everything: Mansell and colleagues say your 'biology (e.g., genes), personality, learning history, traumatic experiences and culture'.

One relevant example here could be those who develop contamination-based OCD during the Covid-19 pandemic. I said previously that the pandemic has been problematic for people who already have this type of OCD: they will have spent years trying to learn that their anxiety about catching contagious illnesses is misplaced, and this will be hugely disrupted by the new global context. But the pandemic could also *trigger* this type of OCD. Some individuals who were vulnerable to having intrusive anxious thoughts will have been on the cusp of developing a disorder when the virus appeared. For these people, legitimate society-wide anxiety around germs and illness could have been their particular 'current context', tipping them in the direction of contamination-based OCD as opposed to, say, GAD.

So according to this transdiagnostic approach to mental illness, which is gaining in popularity, different disorders aren't all that distinct. This doesn't mean we can abandon these diagnostic labels – even if there's lots of overlap, it's still useful to have these somewhat artificial categories. Apart from the practical benefits for treatment and research, some people find a label helpful when faced with the challenge of mental illness, as we shall see. But it serves to remind us that the official list of psychiatric diagnoses is essentially a list of ideas, not a catalogue of biological truth. As American psychiatrist Kenneth Kendler writes:

Imagine turning the clock back ten thousand years and allowing human civilization to again develop agriculture, writing, science, medicine, and, finally, something resembling psychiatry. Then we wait till this psychiatry-like discipline decides to write a diagnostic manual and we get a copy of this manual. We then repeat this experiment 100 times and classify the resulting categories alongside our current DSM-5 and ICD-10. What will we find? My intuition (and those of many with whom I have shared this thought experiment) is that a substantial proportion of our current categories will not be represented reliably in these manuals. Unlike the elements in the periodic table, our current menu of psychiatric disorders would not likely be consistently rediscovered.[23]

Cultural syndromes

The influence of time and place explains the existence of 'cultural syndromes', specific disorders that only crop up in certain places – like *koro*, which is found in diverse ethnic and religious groups in Asia and Africa. This rare disorder is characterised by the acute anxiety that one's penis is shrinking or disappearing. The scientific literature on the topic includes papers describing 'the psychological disappearance of the penis',[24] 'dysmorphic penis image perception'[25] and 'magical penis loss'.[26] This disorder – the name or the symptoms – doesn't appear in the Western world. Others are *reflechi twòp* (thinking too much), which is found only in Haiti,[27] and *Hwa-byung* (rage virus), which is found only in Korea. A Korean review found that, when individuals with *Hwa-byung* were also assessed for DSM disorders, they often met criteria for anger disorders, GAD or depression, although it did not entirely overlap with any of these.[28]

Some of these cultural differences can be explained by 'idioms of distress'[29] – that different ways for expressing distress are considered acceptable in different cultures. In some cultures, for example, it's more acceptable for depression to manifest itself as physical pain. This can be a real problem when it comes to treating and supporting individuals from different cultures, particularly in a service that lacks diversity or sufficient cultural awareness in its staff.

As Kendler points out, the existence of 'cultural syndromes' can hardly be surprising – different cultures conceptualise a lot of things differently, after all. But again, it serves as an important reminder that the current version of the DSM, and Western conceptualisation of mental disorder more broadly, is just *one* way of looking at mental distress. The terms in it are a helpful and often necessary way of packaging mental distress, in a way that allows us to understand and treat it, but we should use them somewhat loosely.

In the previous two chapters we have seen some of the challenges of defining mental illness and how, in some of the DSM, this has led to more experiences being categorised as disorders now than in the past. One might be tempted to conclude that this is why we have been seeing an increase in rates of mental illness: thanks to the expanding DSM, professionals are seeing and diagnosing disorders where previously they did not. But it's not as straightforward as that. As I said, many mental health professionals (especially in the UK) do not rely religiously on specific criteria to reach a diagnosis – many, particularly psychotherapists, don't rely on a diagnosis at all. In addition, the most recent version of the DSM has also contracted or removed some disorders, meaning it hasn't clearly led to higher rates of diagnoses overall. This means that the vertical and horizontal expansion happening in some of the DSM cannot be the whole picture. To understand why we have higher rates of mental illness today, we need to step away from this manual and look more broadly at what else is happening in society. And for that, we need to understand what actually causes mental illness and its symptoms in the first place.

CHAPTER 4

Biology

Found within every living being, DNA is the cookbook for how to make that specific person or creature or plant. Genes, which are segments of DNA, are the individual recipes: they contain instructions for every aspect of how you function. If you could read the microscopic strands of DNA that are found in nearly every cell of your body and compare them with those of any other human, you would find they were very similar: over 99% of our genetic material is the same across all humans.[1] But in less than 1% of our genes, there are subtle differences in the instructions, and this – in genetic terms, at least – is what makes us unique.

Genes shape us by instructing our bodies to make the specific proteins that are responsible for everything that make us who we are – our eye colour, our height, everything to do with how our bodies operate, including our brain: how it is physically structured and how it functions. Genes affect how quickly and readily electrochemical signals are sent and where they are sent, for example – and both of these affect our thoughts, feelings and behaviour. This being the case, it must be that genetics are involved in some capacity in mental illness. But it's difficult to figure out which genes are involved, and what exactly it is that they do.

It's long been established that if one of your first-degree relatives (parents, siblings or children) has a mental disorder, you are more likely to have that disorder yourself. But extra evidence is needed to tell us to what extent this is down to genes specifically, rather than other shared factors or means of inheritance. To determine if genes are involved, scientists turn to twins and adopted children.

Some twins are identical, sharing all their DNA, and some are non-identical, sharing 50% of the DNA just like regular siblings, and this distinction is really useful for working out whether mental illness (or anything else) has a genetic basis. In a twin study, researchers recruit hundreds or thousands of pairs of twins, some identical and some non-identical. They then record all the individuals in the study that have a feature or disorder of interest, like depression, say, and then look to see whether the other twin also has depression. If the likelihood of having a fellow depressed twin is higher in the identical than non-identical twin pairs, then you can draw the conclusion that genetics are involved.

This is because all twins, identical and non-identical, share similar environments – parenting, schooling, family wealth, etc. (Twin studies are based on the assumption that all identical and non-identical twin pairs really do share the same environment, which is imperfect, but works broadly across enough sets of twins.) If the cause of depression was found purely in the environment, you would expect the risk of depression to be the same for *anyone* with a depressed twin, identical or not. But if the disorder has a genetic basis, you would see stronger rates of depression co-occurrence in the identical pairs, because these twins share their environment *and* their genes. And this is exactly what has been found for mental illness: thousands of twin studies have shown that all psychiatric disorders are genetic to some extent. The risk of your twin developing the same mental disorder as you is much higher if you are genetically identical.

The role of genes has also been indicated in adoption studies – and convergence like this across different research methods is always reassuring. With this approach, scientists study children who are being brought up by adoptive parents – i.e. parents with whom they share no genetic material. To continue with the depression example: in these studies, scientists measure levels of depression in biological parents, their adopted-away child, and the child's adoptive parents. The adoption study is a particularly useful design because, as we will see in the next chapter, the genetic risk that our parents hand down to us can be hard to tease apart from the home environment they provide for us. If there is a link between biological parents and their adopted-away children – i.e. if heightened depression in a parent is linked to heightened depression in their biological kids, even when they are raised by someone else – then we can be confident that genetics are contributing. And this is exactly what has been found for a host of psychiatric disorders: the child of a parent with mental illness remains at heightened risk for that disorder themselves, even when they are adopted (this is about relative risk, of course: having a parent with a mental illness is no guarantee that a child will develop it themselves).

Which genes are we talking about?

Thanks to twin and adoption studies, it is undisputed that the risk of mental illness is at least partly influenced by our genes. The trickier bit is working out exactly what genes are involved. Twin and adoption studies tell us that *some* genes are relevant, but they don't tell us which ones. This is important because if researchers are ever going to use genetic information to identify or treat mental illness, they need to know which genes – of the possible 20,000 – are responsible.

Research so far has told us there is not an individual gene that codes for any specific mental illness. There is no 'bipolar disorder gene' or 'bulimia gene'. Instead, mental disorders are *polygenic*: hundreds and possibly even thousands of different genes play a role, with each one conferring a small additional risk for the person. This is not surprising: even for eye colour, there are at least fifteen genes involved. For something as complex as mental illness, where a huge number of cognitive processes, emotions and behaviours are involved, it makes sense that this will involve many genes.

For schizophrenia, 108 specific gene locations have been found to be important, although there are likely to be many more.[2] When a disorder is entirely genetic, genes explain 100% of the risk for that disorder: they fully explain, statistically, why one person develops a disorder while another person doesn't. In schizophrenia, that figure is around 80%. The trouble is, in practice, we don't know many of the *specific* genes that contribute to that risk in schizophrenia: we just know that genes are involved *in general.* Knowing genetic information from the 108 genes identified in the above study allowed the researchers to predict only 10% of the puzzle of why some people develop the disorder and others don't. The other 70% – a large number of other specific genes – are yet to be identified.

Attempts at uncovering the genetic architecture of depression have been even less successful: a 2018 study[3] of over 480,000 individuals identified forty-four potentially relevant genes, and one from 2019[4] of over 1.3 million people found eighty-seven variants to be important – but these accounted for only a fraction of the risk for developing depression. Then another 2019 study (620,000 individuals) found no promising potential gene locations at all.[5] We still have a long way to go.

Even when specific genes have been identified as important, we need to figure out what that gene actually does. This is a mammoth task: we don't know what all 20,000 of our genes are responsible for, or how the activity of all those genes is biologically controlled (the activity of a gene can be turned on or off). This means that even when a specific version of a gene keeps cropping up in people with mental illness, we don't necessarily know the exact role it plays in the disorder. There are exceptions to this: for example, a 2017 study investigating the genetics of anorexia found that a number of genes involved were those responsible for metabolic processes and digestion (like the processes that convert food into energy, or tell us we're hungry).[6] But for many other disorders, the best we know is that a lot of genes are involved. We don't know exactly what it is that they do.

Another complicating factor is that the same genes seem to play a role in lots of different disorders. For example, gene variants that crop up in people with schizophrenia also appear in those with bipolar disorder, even though these are – currently – considered distinct disorders. As US psychiatrist Jordan Smoller has said: 'Our genes don't seem to have read the DSM.'[7] Add to this the complication that many mental illnesses, particularly depression, are heterogeneous: different people with the same disorder may have very different symptoms or different underlying causes for the same symptom. If you recruit a bunch of people with depression to try and identify which gene variants they share, this is going to be a lost cause if their symptoms are caused by different genes. If there are distinct subtypes of depression, each with their own relevant genes, then we will never identify a consistent genetic vulnerability for depression as a whole.

Then there is evidence that the genes that influence your initial risk of a disorder might be different from the genes that determine how the disorder develops or resolves. In 2015 Jean-Baptiste Pingault and colleagues published two studies looking at the genes that contribute to conduct disorder (a pattern of chronic antisocial behaviour) and ADHD.[8] These studies both relied on a longitudinal cohort dataset of over 8,000 pairs of twins – meaning that the influence of specific genes on behavioural problems could be tracked across time. With both disorders, they found that the genes that appeared to influence people's initial risk of developing the disorder were different to the genes that appeared to explain how the disorder played out across time. This adds another layer of complexity when trying to find which genes contribute to specific disorders.

Finally, as we shall see in the next chapter, DNA can only ever account for one's vulnerability to a disorder, not to the disorder itself. You could live your whole life with a genetic susceptibility to mental illness that never actually rears its head. In order for a vulnerability to develop into a disorder, there must be a trigger to set it off. As a result of all these factors, we are a long way from knowing how genetic information could be used for prevention or treatment of mental disorders. As a group of researchers led by Jordan Smoller said: 'The field [of psychiatric genetics] is facing a problem of daunting complexity.'[9] This may all change in time, we're just not there yet.

Mental disorders as brain disorders

In many respects, the brain is the most obvious place to look when trying to understand the biological cause of mental illness. All of our psychology – every thought, emotion and behaviour – is channelled via the workings of our brain. By definition, therefore, all mental disorders would in some sense be brain disorders. In fact, this idea is rather controversial.

In 2015, psychiatrists Thomas Insel (then director of the National Institute of Mental Health in the US) and Bruce Cuthbert published an article about mental illness in the influential journal *Science* titled 'Brain disorders? Precisely'.[10] In the article, they summarise the recent drive from the NIMH to develop 'precision medicine' in psychiatry. Precision medicine is a targeted approach to illness and disease, where biological (or sometimes environmental or lifestyle) differences in patients are identified to create more specified and effective treatments. For example, before a person starts treatment, they could have a blood test to identify which subtype of the disease they have and therefore which treatment is likely to be most effective for them. This is already happening in other areas of medicine such as cancer treatment, and Insel and Cuthbert are arguing (along with many others) that we should now take the same approach to psychiatry – particularly at the level of brain differences. We need to identify the exact neural systems that are disrupted when a person displays certain symptoms or a disorder, they say; mental disorders should be viewed as 'brain circuit disorders'. Then treatment can be 'individualised based on each person's needs and specific neuropathology'. This is all laudable, but it hasn't happened yet – and some researchers argue that it never will.

Networks

Let's start with what we do know. First, we know that brain dysfunctions associated with mental illness are likely to be caused by disruptions not in any one region alone but in *networks*: groups of brain regions that communicate with each other a lot and have a shared general function. As psychologist Deanna Barch wrote in 2013, 'the complexity and range of impairments present in disorders such as schizophrenia are highly unlikely to be due to impairments in a single system, let alone a single brain region'.[11] There are many such networks, but I will describe three here, as the theory of their combined contribution to mental illness was termed the 'triple network model' by neuroscientist Vinod Menon in 2011.[12]

The first is the default mode network (DMN). This collection of regions, including the medial prefrontal cortex and posterior cingulate cortex, fires up during mind wandering – when thoughts pop into your mind when you're meant to be focusing on something else – or as you're otherwise engaging in quiet, reflective thoughts. This kind of thinking almost always involves thoughts about yourself or about other people in your life. If you put a person in a brain scanner and ask them to do nothing – to just rest or reflect on whatever's going through their head – regions in the DMN become activated. If you ask someone to engage in a specific task, like solving a problem or playing a game, activity in these regions dies down, and activity in two other networks, the salience and central executive networks, fires up. The salience network (SN) – which includes the anterior insula and the anterior cingulate cortex – becomes activated when something of potential importance or significance happens. It could be something external – someone's facial expression, a spider in the corner of the room – or internal, like a thought or sensation in the body. In particular, this network alerts us to things that might have emotional significance, both good and bad. The third network, the central executive network (CEN), is involved in high-level cognitive functions, like planning, decision-making, attention and short-term memory. (These are the executive functions that I mentioned in Chapter 3.) These high-level processes are essential for us to navigate our lives effectively moment by moment, day by day, and in the long term – and are often dysfunctional in people with mental illness.

When these three networks function well, information and instructions glide efficiently between them. When we are doing something relaxing or easy – lying in bed in the morning, driving our car or waiting for the bus – our DMN is active, flicking through past memories, thinking about ourselves or other people, musing about the future. Then when we come up against something – someone calls, we open our emails, we see our car is low on petrol – the DMN calms down and the other two networks kick into action. The SN tells us something important has happened: an email from our boss entitled 'urgent', the petrol light is red on the dashboard – and we shift into panic or problem-solving mode. The CEN helps us decide if the issue is important or just a false alarm, and then helps us figure out what to do. We switch off from our daydreaming and juggle through a work problem in our head; we decide who to call or what document to check; we plan to pull off at the next junction. When we are healthy and fully functioning, information is transferred within and between these networks with lightning efficiency and grace.

But across all psychiatric disorders, activity in these networks is disrupted, and this gives rise to problematic symptoms. Take the DMN, for example. There is lots of evidence that this network is dysfunctional in depression. Interestingly, lack of activity isn't the issue here: for people with this disorder, there seems to be *too much* activity and connectivity in the DMN.

The hypothesis is that the hyperactivity may lead to the excessive amounts of self-focused thought and analytic rumination that appears in depression.[13]

The link between SN dysfunction and mental disorder is also logical. If this network isn't working properly, then significance (or excessive significance) will be attached to the wrong thing, and – in concert with a faulty CEN – attention can become 'locked' in an unhelpful place. This has consistently been found in people with anxiety disorders. In particular, hyperactivity in the anterior insula, a key part of the SN, is common in people prone to anxiety. It has been hypothesised that pathological anxiety arises because of this region, in the words of Menon and Lucina Uddin, 'misattributing emotional salience to mundane events' – like a burglar alarm going off in response to a roaming cat.[14]

The exact nature of what the SN latches onto will depend on the disorder – it might be a potential danger in the outside world (specific phobia), or a passing worry in the mind (GAD), or a physical feeling in the body (panic disorder). No wonder this can lead to anxiety: if your brain is telling you to pay attention to a slightly increased heart rate, for example, like an insistent child tugging on your sleeve, it's not surprising that you will focus your attention there, and that you might then feel panicked.

It's not just anxiety disorders. For example, disruption in the SN is also found in schizophrenia.[15] This can mean that individuals with this disorder attribute too much importance to random thoughts or external events. If a person sees something fleetingly in a newspaper or online, most of the time it would just be forgotten about. But imagine if a surge of brain activity happened in the SN at the same time. This could mean that the story or image appears to have huge significance – and this could contribute to delusions, like believing that a celebrity is speaking to you, or that someone wants to do you harm. Similarly, if excessive salience is attributed to a passing thought, this could lead other parts of the brain to interpret that thought as somehow distinctive from other thoughts. This, in turn, could mean it gets 'tagged' as an external voice, leading to an auditory hallucination (a key theory about hearing voices is that they are self-generated thoughts that are misattributed to something or someone external).

Interestingly, a problem can also arise if regions in the SN aren't paying *enough* attention: like the disruption in this network found in autism spectrum disorder (ASD). Hypoactivity in these regions can mean that individuals with ASD don't pay enough attention to social information like facial expressions – which most people experience as highly salient – which then leads to a cascade of difficulties with social behaviour and relationships.[16]

Our healthy psychological functioning is dependent on all these three networks (and others) communicating in a smooth and balanced fashion. When these networks are not working efficiently, we can get stuck: unable to stop ruminating, unable to distract ourselves from an intrusive thought, unable to navigate a social interaction or deal with an unexpected challenge. And once these patterns become established, mental illness can emerge. Unsurprisingly, then, disruption across these brain networks can be seen in virtually every psychiatric disorder.

Intuitively we know that the brain must be involved in mental illness – because it is the seat of our every experience – and this has been supported by the evidence to date. So why do some people not like the 'mental disorders are brain disorders' approach?

Where's the controversy?

Well firstly, there is the importance of external factors – some people think it's wrong to attribute the cause of mental illness to genes and the brain when difficult life circumstances so clearly contribute to people's risk of a disorder, and we explore this in Chapter 5. But there are other issues here. In 2018, the psychologist Denny Borsboom and colleagues published an article entitled 'Brain disorders? Not really', a play on Insel and Cuthbert's title several years prior.[17] In it, they criticise the current widespread enthusiasm for 'explanatory reductionism' in psychiatry. This is the idea that mental disorders can be explained in terms of specific biological dysfunctions, including brain circuits – exactly what Insel and Cuthbert were advocating for. They aren't disputing whether the brain is involved in mental illness. The answer to that question is a confident yes. Instead, Borsboom and colleagues argue that we shouldn't be putting the brain on a pedestal, so to speak: we can't understand mental illness by *only* looking at the brains of people with these disorders, for a number of reasons.

First, the relationship between brain disruptions and psychiatric symptoms is not a one-way street. *Some* of the brain abnormalities we see in people with mental illness will stem from early, genetically driven differences – ones that existed before the symptoms appeared – but not all of them. This is because the brain is also *affected* by the consequences of actually having a mental illness, as it is by all experience. Take anorexia as an example: individuals who go on to develop anorexia often display a certain pattern of psychological traits in childhood, long before the illness begins, like high levels of anxiety and perfectionism – all of which are underpinned by patterns of neurological functioning.[18] These traits will give rise to things like anxiety around body image and a desire to restrict food intake, which are key symptoms of the disorder. But once anorexia has begun, the illness itself will affect the way the brain functions: starvation has a wide-ranging impact on cognitive and neural function, from impaired concentration to increased irritability and depression.[19] As such, you cannot scan the brains of people with anorexia and draw any conclusions about whether the differences you see *caused* the disorder.

You can be more confident about the causal role of brain disruptions by looking at prospective studies. In these studies, large groups of healthy individuals are scanned, and then tracked over time to see which early neural patterns were present in the minority of individuals who went on to develop the disorder. This has happened in depression, for example, where there is evidence of disruptions in the way the brain processes reward, detectable before the onset of the disorder. Reward plays a critical role in our ability to successfully navigate through life – we have to find things like money and food and social interactions pleasurable, because this helps us to engage in productive goal-directed behaviours. As you may remember from Chapter 2, an inability to experience reward (anhedonia) is one of the two key symptoms of depression (the other being low mood). There's evidence that the brain regions that process reward are disrupted *before* depressive symptoms emerge. For example, one 2019 meta-analysis of sixty-eight longitudinal studies found that, in adolescence, a blunted response to reward in a brain region called the striatum predicted subsequent risk of developing depression.[20] Only by conducting these prospective studies can we see which brain disruptions might predate, and therefore perhaps play a causal role in, the onset of the disorder. Otherwise, if we see dysfunctional reward processing in the brains of people who are depressed we could simply be seeing a consequence of having the disorder: depressive symptoms include changes in sleep, for example, which can in turn affect how you process reward.

This is the first issue with the 'mental disorders are brain disorders' idea. Neural processes and mental illness symptoms both affect *each other* together in a continual back-and-forth loop. On top of that, as we'll see in the next chapter, this loop can be triggered and affected by things that are happening outside of the body. So yes, we can see average differences in the brain scans of people caught up in this brain-symptoms-environment loop (i.e. people with mental illness), but that doesn't mean the brain differences seen in these individuals are the sole cause of the disorder, or that the disruptions seen once the illness has taken hold are necessarily the ones that caused it to begin in the first place.

The problem of overlapping disorders

The second difficulty is that, to confidently call mental disorders brain disorders, we ideally need to find some reliable links between specific brain disruptions and the resulting psychological disorder. This hasn't happened: different studies often find different things. For example, some studies have found that the orbitofrontal cortex (OFC; a region involved in reward processing) is significantly larger in patients with anorexia compared to controls, but other studies have found it's significantly smaller.[21] This may be because one of these findings was bogus, or it may be because patients differ from each other: for some people, a larger OFC increases risk for eating disorders; for others, a smaller one does. We can't say for sure. This may come as a surprise, but we don't yet have a clear understanding of how the size of a brain region translates to psychological experience. At the end of a 2015 paper about the neuroscience of OCD, the researchers summarise the field as follows: 'In common with other psychiatric disorders such as bipolar disorder or schizophrenia, neuroimaging studies in OCD are often contradictory and difficult to interpret.'[22] Even though we know intuitively that the brain must give rise to mental illness, identifying consistent abnormalities has been really hard.

Like with the genetic studies, any abnormality or difference found in one disorder is often found in many other disorders too. For example, people with major depressive disorder tend to have a smaller hippocampus than controls, a brain region involved in long-term memory processes. But this can also be seen in people with schizophrenia, PTSD, alcoholism, epilepsy, Alzheimer's[23] ... and even people who exercise less. In other words, knowing that a person has a smaller than average hippocampus isn't much use, and doesn't give us much confidence that a small hippocampus has any special role in depression specifically. Similarly, abnormalities in the three networks I have described have been found in pretty much every psychiatric disorder, and also neurological disorders like dementia and neurodevelopmental disorders like autism and ADHD.

All this means that, as it stands, we can't currently do a brain scan or a blood test and tell you whether someone has depression or schizophrenia or OCD, or even 'any mental illness'. To use the medical parlance, we have no *biomarkers* for most common mental disorders – objective indicators of a medical state that can be observed from outside the patient. In many other areas of medicine, biomarkers from, say, blood tests and tissue samples are essential for diagnosing illnesses and conditions like cancer and diabetes. With most mental illnesses, there is no such test. We diagnose disorders entirely on the basis of the patient's symptoms, either self-reported or (for children) reported by their parents or teachers. If we know already who has a disorder and who doesn't, we can look at brain scans from the two groups of people and we can detect some average differences in the way the brain is structured or functions (though these differences are often not consistent across studies and the same disruptions are found in many different disorders). But it doesn't work the other way round: we can't look at a single person's brain scan and say whether or not they have a mental illness. The psychologist Eiko Fried summed it up like this: 'The fact of the matter is that, despite many decades of considerable research efforts into uncovering underlying biological mechanisms, we have not identified specific and reliable markers for many of the most prevalent mental disorders.'[24]

The hunt for biomarkers may just be a matter of time and money. Part of the lack of success so far can certainly be linked to funding. According to the MQ mental health research charity, between 2014 and 2017 an average of £124 million was spent on mental health research per year in the UK – an average of £9 for each person with mental illness. By contrast, £612 million per year was spent on cancer research over the same period, which translates to £228 per person affected – twenty-five times more than for mental health.[25] To crack the question of biomarkers, we may just need more money to conduct more research. The advances in cancer and HIV research, for example, were made only once those fields were funded properly.

With more money could come bigger sample sizes (ideally with data shared across different research groups, for maximum efficiency), which would mean more reliable data and more chance to detect subtle effects and differences. Money would allow researchers to track these participants longitudinally, to see the relationship between brain differences and symptoms across time. It would mean better-designed studies, like more refined tasks for individuals to carry out in brain scanners, which can home in on very specific psychological processes. Finally, more funding could mean better-quality equipment, like brain scanners that can detect finer-grained detail with greater precision and sensitivity. All of this is now starting to happen, as society and funding bodies start to recognise the importance of mental health, but it's early days yet.

It's also possible that, in trying to isolate mental illness biomarkers in the brain, researchers are barking up the wrong tree. As I've already implied, the brain doesn't sit on a shelf in a jar of formaldehyde, entirely disconnected from its body or external environment. What may be more fruitful than trying to find differences in the brain alone, then, is to look at the brain in context. As we'll see in the next chapter, vulnerabilities in someone's brain might only be important or apparent when they interact with that person's bigger story and what has happened to them. Some people even argue that we should *stop* channelling more money into looking at the brain. The psychiatrist David Kingdon, for example, said this in 2020: 'Is it not time for research to refocus resource and expertise away from the laboratory and onto these more relevant psychological and social sciences and research into clinical practice, public health and service delivery? ... In terms of emphasis, isn't listening to patients' perceptions of causation [of their mental disorder] more likely to provide insights rather than looking down a microscope?'[26]

I would argue that we need both: we cannot understand how the brain gives rise to mental illness without thinking about the environment in which it sits, but the reverse is also true. As we're about to see, the environment is also important – but its impact will depend on your specific biological make-up. Which brings us to our next question: what happens outside the body that increases our risk of mental illness?

CHAPTER 5

Environment

As the poet Philip Larkin famously explained, our parents, whether they intend to or not, can have a negative influence on us. From the moment we are conceived right through to our teenage years and beyond, our parents' choices and behaviours affect who we are and how we develop. So when we think about the effect of the environment – anything we experience in the outside world – on mental illness, parenting is a good place to start.

A host of parenting behaviours are associated with an increased risk of later mental illness. Of course, outright abuse is harmful for a child – we'll get to that in a moment – but a number of other more 'subtle' parenting habits are also linked to later mental health problems in children. These include rejection (defined in the academic literature as the tendency for parents to criticise and disapprove of the child), control (the tendency for parents to excessively regulate their children's activities and provide overbearing advice and instructions about how the child should think or feel), overprotection (excessive physical contact, infantilising, and preventing the child from trying age-appropriate risk-taking and independent behaviour), and a lack of warmth and affection. Studies have found that children whose parents frequently treat them in these ways are more likely to develop a mental illness later in life.

On the face of it, this is clear evidence that the environment affects your risk of mental illness. But when it comes to parenting – as with many things in this chapter – separating environmental from biological factors is tricky, to say the least. Provided you were brought up by your biological parents, the people parenting you are *also* the people who gave you your genes. The parents of a child who ultimately develops depression are likely *themselves* to be vulnerable to depressive symptoms or possibly to have been actively depressed while bringing up their child. Parents who are prone to depression might be exhausted, irritable, lacking confidence and trapped in a spiral of their own thoughts, leaving them with fewer emotional and physical resources for parenting. This might therefore make them less warm, for example, or more likely to reject their child.

When it comes to mental illness, parents can therefore give you a double whammy of risk. Parents give you their genes, but by virtue of the very same genes, they can also parent you in certain ways that make you more vulnerable. These two things – vulnerable genetics and suboptimal parenting – are tied together, in a non-random way. This is known as *gene-environment correlation*, and it makes it harder to work out the relative contributions of biology and the outside world to our mental health.

These correlations don't just apply to mental illness, of course. Parents who are intellectually curious, for example, will pass on a genetic predisposition to be that way but they will also, if they can afford it, provide an environment – a house full of books, trips to museums – that will foster and encourage that trait. If the child ends up being intellectually curious too, it's hard to distinguish how much that's down to the curiosity genes and how much is down to the bookish environment.

Parenting and anxiety

Imagine a mother and her eight-year-old son, both of whom have social anxiety disorder. (Dads are important too, of course, but much of the research on parenting has been conducted with mothers, usually because they have been more available and willing to participate.) If we want to understand why the son has developed the disorder, we need first to recognise that, since his mum also has it, she may well have passed on genes that elevated his risk. But her own disorder might also have affected his environment in the following ways.

When they attend get-togethers, for example, such as neighbourhood barbecues or school socials or birthday parties, she might act in ways that are typical of those who experience this disorder, such as being quiet or getting upset. Or she might avoid some situations altogether because she finds them too difficult. In the psychological parlance, she 'models' that being anxious, distressed and avoidant is the normal way to behave in social situations. Modelling can of course be positive – it's one of the key ways we learn how to interact with people and the world. But modelling of this sort is an established way in which problematic behaviours can be transferred from one generation to the next. Similarly, aggressive parents might model that shouting is a normal way to deal with conflict; parents with eating disorders might model a dislike or disgust of high-calorie food.

But back to our social anxiety example: the anxious mother might also say certain things about social events – how much she doesn't want to attend them or how much she doesn't want to host people at home – that inadvertently send a message to the child that social events are scary and difficult. And because she believes these situations are difficult, she might step in to try to help her son in social situations, or protect him from experiencing social challenges like playing with new children or joining an after-school club. This is an understandable instinct – to protect her child from situations that she herself finds harmful and scary. But because he has fewer opportunities to practise social skills in these environments and learn that they are not so bad, this overprotectiveness might actually contribute to his own anxiety, making these situations harder for him to deal with and ultimately increasing his risk of developing social anxiety disorder. And this is what the research suggests.

In one longitudinal study published in 2000, just over 1,000 fourteen-to-seventeen-year-olds, and their parent (usually the mother) took part in clinical interviews – independently – to assess any potential mental disorder.[1] The adolescents also completed a questionnaire about their mother's parenting behaviours. Around twenty months later, the participants were all interviewed again. The researchers found that maternal social anxiety disorder (called social phobia in the study) was strongly associated with subsequent social anxiety disorder in their children. Across all participants, parental overprotection (and rejection) was also associated with later social anxiety disorder in the adolescents.

Of course, plenty of people who suffer from depression, anxiety disorders and other mental illnesses are wonderful parents; plenty of them don't have children with the same difficulties. Equally, lots of people reject or criticise or overprotect their children in the absence of any resulting mental illness. This is just about relative risk. If you have a history of mental illness, you *can* pass this onto your child, in part because of your genes, and in part because your own psychological tendencies can affect the way you parent.

I write this with a great deal of compassion because I know that people with a history of these difficulties often feel torn about having a child. The writer Esmé Weijun Wang, quoted at the end of Chapter 2 in relation to the DSM-5, writes movingly on this topic in her book, *The Collected Schizophrenias*. When people ask her if she wants children, she says she talks vaguely about having a genetic disorder and not wanting to pass it on, and of the impact that her medication might have on a foetus. When she says this, people often ask if she has considered adoption, and this is how she wants to respond: 'What I want to say is I have schizoaffective disorder. I was psychotic for half of 2013, and I could be psychotic at any moment. I don't want to put a child through having me as a mother.'[2]

Having a mental illness should never preclude anyone from having a child or the chance to be a loving and supportive parent. What I'm saying is that having a baby is always a big decision, and it can be even harder for some people who have, or have had, a mental illness.

The role of the child

So far we've focused on how parenting can contribute to mental illness, but there are two people in a parent–child relationship, and the child can affect the way they are parented. The relationship between parents' genes and the environment they create for their children is an example of a *passive* gene-environment correlation, but there are also *evocative* gene-environment correlations. These occur when, as a result of a child's genes, that child consistently elicits certain reactions from the people around them, including their parents.

Children who are anxious will often flat out refuse to do things, like going to sleepovers or swimming lessons or school, or experience a lot of distress in these situations. Knowing that your child is going to be anxious in certain situations could unsurprisingly lead to a parent feeling more protective over them. A depressed child or teenager who is always irritable and despondent may elicit a frustrated reaction from his parents. Children who consistently show a lack of empathy or guilt (known as *callous-unemotional* traits, a potential precursor to adult psychopathy) often have parents who are less warm. Maybe this lack of warmth contributed to the child's tendencies in the first place, but it might also be hard to be consistently affectionate to a child or adolescent who is deceitful, manipulative and cold. In other words, again, a child's genes are linked in a non-random way to their environment. This is another reason why we cannot look at the effects of biology in isolation.

When parents do contribute to a person's risk of mental illness, the way they do this isn't straightforward. It's partly genetic and it's partly parenting behaviour, which are linked, and the child's own temperament can sometimes lead to problematic responses from their carers. Children and adolescents with mental health problems can become embroiled in a complicated and dysfunctional loop of interactions with their parent, who might also be showing the same propensities as their child; many of them will be trying their best in challenging circumstances.

Child maltreatment

Any sympathy for parents crumbles to dust when we move beyond tried-their-best, occasional limitations and into something much darker. When thinking about the environmental causes of mental illness, we need to address one of the most damaging things that can happen to a person: child abuse.

Child maltreatment – the broader term – is divided by professionals into four categories. *Physical abuse* is any non-accidental injury resulting from deliberate actions, and can include beating, kicking or anything else that causes physical harm. *Sexual abuse* is any sexual activity with a child. It can involve physical contact with the child, or not – such as making a child watch sex acts or pornography. *Emotional* (or *psychological*) *abuse* is an inappropriate emotional response to a child's needs, and can include insulting, mocking or ignoring them. Finally, *neglect* refers to an absence of appropriate caring of a child, like not providing them with adequate food or clothing, or not taking them to the doctor when needed. The different types of maltreatment often occur alongside each other, and typically happen within the home. Most of the time, it is parents who are abusing their own children. One 2007 study from the US found that in 80.1% of all cases, the abuse was carried out by one or both of the child's own parents (most commonly – in 38.7% of all cases – the abuse was enacted by a mother alone).[3]

It can be shocking to learn how prevalent such abuse is. One 2015 meta-analysis reviewed 244 publications from around the world and found that, across genders, 22.6% of children had experienced physical abuse, 12.8% sexual abuse, 36.3%

emotional abuse, and 17.4% neglect.[4] In the US, at least 1,500 children die a year as a result of maltreatment.[5] If these numbers seem particularly high to you, then this is just evidence of how hidden a problem this is. One year when I taught a lecture on this topic, two students (out of a class of about forty) asked to be excused in advance, for personal reasons.

It's well established that experiencing child maltreatment can be devastating for a person's psychological development, increasing the risk of mental illness decades into the future. The majority of this research has been conducted in relation to sexual abuse, and this has shown that a history of such abuse is associated with increased rates of anxiety disorders, depression, eating disorders, PTSD, sleep disorders and suicide attempts.[6] The body of research on non-sexual maltreatment is smaller, but shows that this type of abuse is also associated with increased rates of (at least) depression, drug use and suicide attempts.[7] Moreover, mental disorders in people who have experienced maltreatment run a particularly severe course. These individuals tend to have more severe, persistent and recurrent symptoms, which develop earlier; they are more likely to have more than one disorder; and they are less likely to respond to treatment.[8]

To understand why maltreatment increases risk in the way that it does, we must first step outside the home to consider environmental risk factors for mental illness in a wider sense.

Stressful life events

The simple fact is that if particularly difficult, stressful things happen to you, either as a one-off or as a chronic problem, you have a greater risk of mental illness, self-harm and suicide. There are the monumental events: being a victim of war, terrorist attack, natural disaster or displacement – the events that clearly fall under that tricky definition of 'trauma'. And then there are the more mundane hardships: bullying, bereavement, divorce, redundancy; the quiet, chronic stressors of poverty, disadvantage, disability and illness. Of course, many people will be exposed to multiple stressful events, often at the same time, and they all play an important role in the onset of almost all psychiatric disorders, not just PTSD. For example, one study found that at least 80% of individuals with panic disorder experienced at least one stressful life event in the year preceding the onset of the disorder.[9] Another found that if you experience an 'unexpected, negative, very important life event', your risk of subsequently developing GAD triples;[10] for those who already have GAD but have recovered, experiencing a significant life event increases the risk of relapse.[11] Stressful life events commonly precede an episode of depression.

This shouldn't come as a surprise. If you have experience of mental illness yourself, you can likely think about specific stressors that were happening, in the long or short term, before your symptoms started. Or you may recognise the phenomenon in someone else: if someone you love has had a period of mental illness, you may be able to link it to a trigger, something difficult that was going on in their life, big or small. (This 'big or small' bit is critical: as we'll see, and as I said when we talked about PTSD, stressful events are hard to objectively define.) So what are the mechanisms by which stress increases our risk?

Stress affects the way our body and brain functions in several ways. One is via a set of biological processes that occur along the hypothalamus-pituitary-adrenalin (HPA) axis. When the HPA axis is triggered by stress, it sets off a cascade of communication from the hypothalamus to the pituitary gland (both in the brain) to the adrenal glands that sit on top of your kidneys. This causes the release of cortisol, a stress hormone. Cortisol is essential when dealing with short-term threat: it increases your blood pressure and makes your heart pump faster; it increases glucose in the blood to give you more energy. The problem arises when this HPA axis is triggered too often, or when the stress is so severe or chronic that this system doesn't have a chance to dampen down, or when the system gets 'stuck' on high alert even once the stress has ended. 'In PTSD,' says psychiatrist Bessel van der Kolk, 'the body continues to defend against a threat that belongs in the past.'[12] With a prolonged stress response, the effect of cortisol and other biological processes can affect your brain's capacity to process information and affect the health of your entire body, even paving the way to an early grave.

Our focus here will be on the impact that stress has on our psychological functioning. This is inevitably underscored by changes in the brain, and these are partly a result of this HPA axis overactivation. But instead of focusing on the minutiae of the biological effects of stress, we will examine the effects as they manifest themselves in our thoughts, feelings and behaviour – our psychology – and how that can increase our risk of mental illness.

Threat processing

One route is that chronic stress affects the way we process threatening information. This is linked to the brain's salience network I mentioned in the previous chapter, which detects potential dangers in our surroundings. People exposed for prolonged periods to high-stress environments become very attuned to threats – regions in their salience network, like the anterior insula and anterior cingulate cortex, become very good at their job. This makes sense: for children who are being maltreated or bullied, anyone who lives in an area with high levels of community violence, or who is being persecuted, or at war, hypersensitivity to threat may be essential to survival in such dangerous or unpredictable environments.

The trouble is we struggle to live in a constant state of such high alert, and some people continue to show this hyperactive threat response, even well after they have left the dangerous environment. In one 2011 study, UK children with and without a history of maltreatment had their brains scanned while looking at faces showing different emotions.[13] The children with a history of maltreatment were no longer in the abusive environment, for example through adoption, but the experience had left its mark. When looking at the photos of angry faces, they showed more activation in their amygdala – a region critical in processing threat and fear – compared to control children. The more violence they had experienced at home, the more activation they had in this area. This was one of a series of studies that contributed to the 'latent vulnerability hypothesis' put forward by psychologists Eamon McCrory and Essi Viding to help explain why being maltreated can increase future risk of mental illness.[8] The idea is that neural and psychological processes are 'calibrated' to the dangerous environment at the time – they are necessary and even useful in that context – but they come with a cost in the long term.

The way we see things

Stressful life events also contribute to mental illness because they can affect the way we view ourselves, the world and other people. One 2003 study – of 7,322 adult twins in Virginia – looked at the specific features of life events that were linked to subsequently developing depression and GAD.[14] They found that events in which a *loss* had occurred (like a death or divorce) were more likely to trigger both depression and GAD than events that didn't involve loss. Events that involved *humiliation* – things that 'directly devalue an individual in a core role' also predicted depression. Life events with high levels of *danger* predicted the onset of GAD, and high levels of *entrapment* (a sense that circumstances would persist or get worse, and that there was no chance for resolution) predicted the onset of combined depression and GAD. Of course, you can imagine that some events might fall into more than one of these categories – if your partner leaves you for someone else you experience loss and humiliation; if you have been displaced as a victim of war then you will potentially experience all four.

Humiliation may be particularly relevant when it comes to understanding why bullying can contribute to later mental illness. Though often considered a two-person interaction, bullying is typically a group activity, as it takes place in front of an audience – who rarely intervene – and this is humiliating. It is also common now for incidents of bullying to be recorded and shared online, which can amplify the humiliation. In an attempt to understand why they are being victimised, those who are continually being mocked, insulted and attacked by others, particularly those who are young, whose sense of self is new and fragile, often come to believe that they must deserve such treatment. A sad fact is that children who are abused at home are also more likely to be bullied at school; some children are therefore constantly around people who treat them badly.[15] If other people repeatedly behave like you don't deserve love and respect and you don't matter, it's not difficult to see why you might internalise that message. Low self-worth of this sort is a key feature of several mental illnesses, particularly depression and eating disorders.

Stressful life events can also affect how you feel about other people: whether you think others are ultimately trustworthy and safe, or whether you think others are out to trick and hurt you. Even a single event such as being dumped or cheated on can affect a person's ability to trust future partners, limiting their ability to form the very relationships that can shield us from depression and unhappiness. Being repeatedly let down or betrayed by others can undermine a person's ability to form any secure relationships at all. Borderline personality disorder, for example, is characterised by chaotic and mistrustful social behaviour – and these individuals are often found to have had abusive early experiences.[16] A refugee who has been persecuted at home and continues to be marginalised in a new country will have had a string of experiences that very legitimately make her feel like the world is unsafe and people cannot be trusted. In fact, paranoia – a key symptom of psychosis – is consistently elevated in marginalised populations.[17] No wonder: these individuals feel like they are being targeted because in many cases, they really are. It's easy to see how this could escalate into potentially misplaced and excessive paranoid delusions.

I could go on, but the bottom line is this: stressful life events affect the way you process reward, your sense of hope for the future, your ability to regulate your emotions, your memory, your capacity to process new information ... essentially all the processes that, as we've seen so far, can put you at risk for developing mental illness. But we are still missing something important. Experiencing stress, trauma and disadvantage – even a hell of a lot of it – doesn't guarantee that anyone will develop a mental illness. Something else is needed too.

Stress doesn't affect everyone in the same way

The majority of people will experience at least one major difficult event in their lifetime. A study from 1998 of over 2,000 adults in Detroit aged between eighteen and forty-five investigated how many of them had experienced at least one 'traumatic' event in their life, based on the definition in the DSM-IV – any event that involved actual or threatened death or serious injury, either experienced directly or witnessed or experienced by a family member or other 'close associate'.[18] So in this study, traumatic events would include being violently mugged or learning that a close relative or friend had been seriously injured in an accident. The researchers found that 89.6% of participants had experienced at least one of these events. In fact, the average number of traumatic events experienced in the participants' lives to date was 5.3 events for men and 4.3 for women.

And yet, of all these participants, only 9.2% of them met criteria for PTSD in response to one of the traumatic events (this was assessed by clinical interview, using DSM-IV criteria). The majority of people who are exposed to awful events and circumstances actually don't develop a mental disorder.

This probably comes as no surprise. Many of us know someone who has been handed a disproportionate series of challenges but who shows no signs of mental illness. Most of us at some point in our lives grieve and suffer and are upset in the face of hardship but do not experience a prolonged disorder. Studies show that stressful experiences increase our risk of mental illness, but plainly not everyone who experiences life stress will develop a disorder. What does this tell us? Just as biological factors appear to be necessary but not sufficient to explain the onset of mental illness, so too are the environmental factors we have just discussed.

Instead, *both* are required: the predisposition that increases your risk and the trigger to kick it off. Psychologist Danielle Dick sums up the relationship between an individual's genetics, external stress and depression as follows: 'When life stressors are encountered, genetically vulnerable individuals are more prone to developing depression, whereas in the absence of life stressors, these individuals may be no more likely to develop depression. In essence, it is only when adverse environmental conditions are experienced that the genes "come online".'[19]

Importantly, the external stress that triggers a mental disorder need not be anything monumental – especially if you're already susceptible to these problems. In my case, it was a health concern that triggered my first episode of depression. In the months and years leading up to that summer, I had experienced some chronic physical health problems. (For me, as with many others, physical and mental health have always been closely intertwined, so much so that I don't think the distinction between the two labels is particularly meaningful.) A few days before I went on holiday, I saw a specialist who said, in a pretty offhand manner, that my symptoms might be caused by a long-term condition that could cause ongoing pain. It was exactly this that I was thinking about on holiday, as I was walking back to the apartment that day: I was thinking about that potential diagnosis and its implications. For many people, this unconfirmed risk and its possible consequences would have been manageable. But for me, it came at a moment when I was already fragile, so it didn't take much. That appointment – and then going away before I could get the results – was the final flick that caused my psychological house of cards to collapse.

A crucial factor that helps determine our relative resilience to stress are the strategies we engage in to manage its effects. We all have different levels of stress we can tolerate before we get overwhelmed partly because we have different ways of *coping* with that stress – and some of them are more likely than others to lead to later mental health problems or disorders. Broadly, there are two coping styles: active and passive. Active coping strategies include looking for solutions to problems, seeking social support, and talking about difficult events with trusted other people. A passive coping style is more problematic, and is all about avoiding dealing with the stress. It includes rumination (dwelling on the problem), suppressing thoughts about it, and self-medicating with alcohol or other substances.

There is now a large body of research showing that people who engage in passive coping in the aftermath of a trauma or stressful event are more likely to develop a mental illness, and not just PTSD. Researchers looking at the psychological risk factors for depression and anxiety disorders said these included signs of passive coping – 'attempts to alter, avoid, or control emotional responding'.[20] This is often helpful in the short term – it can protect us from overwhelming feelings of anxiety and distress – but in the long term, it impedes our ability to process what has happened to us.

The way people interpret and evaluate stressful events – called 'cognitive appraisal' or just 'appraisal' – is also important. The same experience can be evaluated very differently by different people. Those who engage in positive reappraisal – recognising that something wasn't their fault, for example, or finding benefits in difficult situations – are less likely to be badly affected. But the more you *subjectively* view something as threatening, harmful, out of your control, and leading to a loss, the more at risk you are of developing long-term psychological difficulties. Miranda Olff and colleagues, PTSD researchers from the Netherlands, say that subjective appraisals of events 'may explain why someone develops PTSD after stressful, but seemingly non-catastrophic events (e.g. a divorce), whereas others never develop PTSD after a seemingly horrific trauma (e.g. capture and torture)'.[21] These propensities won't appear for the first time when disaster strikes: we all show long-standing patterns in how we respond to difficulties, and they rear their head whenever a challenge or hardship arises.

The Covid-19 pandemic is a perfect example of this. Of course, some people were objectively affected much more deeply by the pandemic: those who lost their jobs, or became seriously ill, or who were already in poverty. But there was also considerable variety in how the virus *subjectively* affected people. A study published in July 2020 reported that some individuals showed a particularly extreme psychological response in the early months of the pandemic, symptoms like nightmares, intrusive thoughts and compulsive checking. The authors referred to this collection of symptoms as 'Covid stress syndrome'.[22] Importantly, a second study showed that people with a pre-existing anxiety disorder were more likely to show high levels of this Covid-related stress.[23]

None of this is to say that people who don't develop a disorder in the aftermath of difficult events should be viewed as stronger or superior somehow. If a person is sensitive to the effects of stress, there will be a whole host of factors why this is, and a lot of them are bottom-up, biological factors over which they have little control. Their brains, for example, might be hyperresponsive to noticing and reacting to potential threat. This hypersensitivity might then trigger a release of stress hormones via the HPA axis, causing a cascade of stress and panic throughout the body. All of this can mean that stressful experiences are programmed into the brain as particularly vivid memories. The fact that stress is so frightening in the moment, and remembered so vividly, could then – very understandably – make a person more worried about stressful things happening in the future. So the way we respond to stress is a complex combination of our biology, psychological tendencies and upbringing – not a question of moral character. Indeed, it is those of us who are disposed to react badly to stress, rather than those who shrug it off easily, who are arguably the braver and more impressive, but any kind of moral judgement is out of place. We just have different minds and bodies that respond differently to the outside world.

Biology and environment as two warring explanations

Not all mental illnesses are triggered by events in the outside world. For some people, the trigger will be internal – the biological changes of puberty, for example (more on that in the next chapter). But in many cases, symptoms are often set off by some hardship or suffering in the outside world – which tells us that extreme distress, and other symptoms, are often simply your body and mind saying that you're under more stress than you can bear. This has led some people to question whether the label 'disorder' or 'illness' is entirely appropriate. To take some extreme examples, if a person has been tortured or kidnapped or seen their friends die in front of them, triggering symptoms of 'PTSD', should that reaction really be framed as a 'disorder?' The Austrian neurologist and psychiatrist Viktor Frankl, who survived Nazi concentration camps that killed his father, mother, brother and wife, said: 'An abnormal reaction to an abnormal situation is normal behaviour.'[24] Similarly, the psychiatrist R. D. Laing, a prominent early critic of the medicalisation of mental distress, said that insanity was 'a perfectly rational adjustment to an insane world'.[25] Of schizophrenia, he said, 'The experience and behaviour that gets labelled schizophrenic is a special strategy that a person invents in order to live in an unliveable situation.'[26] More recently, the psychologist Lucy Johnstone argues that when someone is distressed, instead of asking 'What is wrong with you?' we should ask, 'What has happened to you?'[27]

Personally, I don't think we should drop the label of mental illness or disorder altogether. People are made prisoner by panic attacks, hopelessness and surging mania; become consumed by terrifying delusions and hallucinations; starve and injure themselves; and harm the relationships and jobs that they need because of overwhelming compulsions. Calling these 'illnesses' or 'disorders' usefully captures the extremity of the psychological pain involved, and how disabling it can all be. But because stress plays the role that it does in causing mental illness, some people are vehemently opposed to the notion that mental illness should be thought of as a *biological* disruption in the brain; they argue we should not use the term mental *illness* at all because this locates the problem in the individual rather than the outside world.

In 2018, for example, the writer Johann Hari published an extract from his book *Lost Connections: Uncovering the real causes of depression – and the unexpected solutions*,[28] entitled 'Is everything you think you know about depression wrong?' In it, he argued that it's wrong and unfair to say that depression, which he suffers from himself, is the result of biological problems. Instead, he says, depression is a response to genuine difficulty and loss in the real world. He ends the article with this: 'If you are depressed and anxious, you are not a machine with malfunctioning parts. You are a human being with unmet needs. The only real way out of our epidemic of despair is for all of us, together, to begin to meet those human needs – for deep connection, to the things that really matter in life.'[29]

The ensuing discussion around Hari's book shows how fraught this topic is. Less than forty-eight hours after the above extract was published, neuroscientist Dean Burnett wrote his own article in the same publication, entitled 'Is everything Johann Hari knows about depression wrong?'

There were several reasons why Hari touched such a nerve. First, Burnett said, Hari presented the idea that life stress is important in mental illness as though it was a brand-new idea. Actually, as we've seen, researchers have recognised this for decades. But more importantly, Burnett and others were concerned because Hari was implying that the cause of depression lies *exclusively* in the outside world, and has nothing to do with people's biology – that they are not 'machines with malfunctioning parts'. The concern was that, by extension, he was saying that the treatment shouldn't be biological either. He doesn't explicitly tell people to avoid antidepressants or stop taking these drugs, but he said, 'At the moment, we offer depressed people a menu with only one option on it' (i.e. medication) and emphasised that people should consider other options. This also riled people, because it's not true that people with depression are only offered drugs. The concern in the academic community was that Hari's emphasis on social causes, and dismissal of the biological, could be irresponsible and misinterpreted.

But I'm not sure there needs to be a battle at all. People on both sides of this debate can be quick to portray the other as extreme: those who argue that mental illness stems from disruption in the brain are said to be dismissing the outside world as irrelevant; those who argue that mental illness derives from life circumstances find it insulting and insensitive that the person's brain is being blamed. In fact, the evidence to date shows that individual vulnerability *and* external factors are both relevant when it comes to mental illness.

The network theory of mental disorders

The most useful theory of mental illness I've come across, which ties together everything said thus far, is the network theory of mental disorders. It was first introduced by Dutch psychologist Denny Borsboom in 2017 and for me, it's the best explanation of what mental illness really 'is'.[30] Borsboom and colleagues argue, as others have done, that it is no use trying to understand mental illness on a single level of explanation like biology or psychology, or to give particular priority to one level over another. Instead, they describe mental illnesses as 'constellations of properties (defined at different theoretical levels) that hang together because they are connected by a diverse set of mechanisms'. Let's break down what this means.

Central to this idea is that biological, psychological and environmental aspects of mental illness exist in an interacting web, all influencing one another. Borsboom and colleagues argue that symptoms don't arise only from biological dysfunction. Instead, they say that symptoms can *cause and influence each other*. Let's take the example of insomnia and fatigue, two symptoms of major depression that often co-occur. They argue that it's probably not the case that a pathological process gives rise to insomnia and fatigue separately. Instead, it's more likely that something triggered the insomnia (e.g. a bereavement, stress at work), and then that in itself caused the person to be fatigued. This could then set off a chain reaction of other depressive symptoms. For example, being tired can cause low mood, and if you're not getting anything done because of the tiredness and low mood, that could cause a drop in self-esteem. In other words, when one symptom gets activated, that symptom in itself can trigger others. In the example above, we don't need to look for initial causes for anything other than the insomnia. They argue that mental disorders are therefore networks of symptoms that directly influence each other. In this way, a disorder 'grows out of a network of symptom–symptom relations'.

The network theory suggests that what initially triggers the mental illness might be something outside of the person, like losing a loved one, but it could also be a biological trigger. Maybe the person developed sleep apnoea (which causes difficulty breathing when sleeping), and that started the insomnia. Or to take a different example: someone might have a brain dysfunction that causes auditory sensations within the brain to be labelled as external voices, which could trigger the experience of an auditory hallucination (hearing voices). The catastrophic misinterpretation of bodily symptoms could lead to a panic attack that then leads to panic disorder; the insufficient ability to manage unwanted thoughts could lead to excessive worry.

As we'll see in the next chapter, the trigger could even just be 'growing up'. For example, schizophrenia typically appears in late adolescence, which has led many researchers to hypothesise that it's the neural and hormonal changes inherent in adolescence that may trigger the start of the disorder for some young people.[31] Here, it is internal biological changes that are the spark, setting off the chain of symptoms that eventually turn into a fire.

What I find particularly interesting about the network theory is that the authors say this cascade of interactions between symptoms can then become *self-sustaining*. In other words, the ties between the symptoms become sufficiently strong that the network sustains its own activation, maintaining the disorder even if the initial trigger has calmed down or disappeared. In this way, Borsboom and colleagues say that to have a disorder means 'to be trapped in a stable state of a self-sustaining symptom network'.

We all like simple explanations. When a person is struck down with mental illness, they want to know why it's happened to them. It also doesn't help that people with anxiety disorders and depression, in particular, are naturally prone to analyse and ruminate. But the truth is that there is no simple explanation for anyone's disorder or distress. We are all a bundle of hundreds of layers of explanation – some biological and some environmental – and those layers all interact with each other. You can start off on a very grand scale, thinking about how the society you live in has affected you, or your friends and family, or you can also zoom in very close, into your psychology, your brain, your DNA. But you may be better off just accepting that it *all* played a role: the factors that led to your disorder are as many and varied as we are.

At the end of Chapter 1, I suggested there may be many factors behind the reported rise in rates of mental illness. In the four chapters that followed, we saw that the symptoms of mental illness are not always easily distinguishable from the 'normal' thoughts, feelings and behaviours involved in everyday living – and that the official demarcation between the two has generally shifted in favour of milder problems. We have seen the biological and environmental factors that can contribute to symptoms, and examined what mental illness really is: a suite of interrelated, mutually enhancing symptoms and difficulties that, once established, might even be said to cause itself. But before we draw all these threads together and consider how they might explain what is happening in society right now, there remain two topics that need to be addressed directly: why the conversation is so often focused on young people, and the role of social media. We will tackle each of them in turn.

CHAPTER 6

Adolescence

If you could relive your adolescence, would you? A few years ago, I went to a talk by psychologist Stella Chan, who researches adolescent depression. She asked the audience this question, and we tapped in our answer using electronic audience participation on our phones. She showed us that 60% of the audience said no, 21% said they weren't sure, and only 19% said yes. Objectively, adolescence might seem like a great period of life – you're comparatively fit and healthy, you're less likely to have caring responsibilities, you have a world of options ahead of you – but in reality, adolescence is a turbulent, challenging time. If given the choice, few people would want to go through it again.

At the start of this book, we saw that the public conversation around mental health often focuses on young people. This is for good reason. If you're ever going to develop a mental illness, more likely than not, it will start in your adolescent years. This finding is based on two big studies conducted in the 2000s. The first was published in 2003 by a group of psychologists in New Zealand led by Julia Kim-Cohen.[1] It was one of many papers published from a cohort study – a type of study in which participants sign up to being tracked across time, often several decades, periodically providing the researchers with data about themselves. This particular cohort was the Dunedin Multidisciplinary Health and Development

Study, which tracked just over 1,000 people, born in 1972 and 1973, for nearly thirty years. Six times, between the ages of eleven and twenty-six, participants took part in interviews that asked about possible psychiatric symptoms. These interviews were conducted by trained interviewers, although not necessarily people with clinical expertise.

To investigate the question of when mental illness begins, these researchers looked first at the most recent psychiatric interviews, conducted when the participants were twenty-six years old. Data was available for 976 people. The researchers looked at how many participants had a diagnosable mental illness at this age, according to the latest DSM criteria. They chose to look at seven categories of disorder: anxiety disorders, depression, mania, eating disorders, substance use disorder, schizophrenia, and antisocial personality disorder. For the individuals with a diagnosable mental illness at twenty-six, the researchers then looked back at what these people had said during their previous five psychiatric interviews, between the ages of eleven and twenty-one. The researchers found that the majority of these participants – 82% – already met criteria for the mental illness at one of the previous time points. Most importantly, 74% of them met this diagnosis when they were eighteen, and 50% met the diagnosis by the time they were fifteen. This was a landmark finding, because it indicated that the majority of mental illness actually starts very young indeed, in the teenage years.

The second study was led by Ronald Kessler in the United States in 2005.[2] It's useful to look at this study alongside Kim-Cohen's study as it takes a slightly different approach. In the US study, interviews were used again, but participants weren't recruited as children. At the start of the study, participants (9,282 of them) were already adults, aged eighteen to sixty. They all lived in the Michigan area, and the sample was nationally representative (there was an accurate range of age, sex, ethnicity and social economic status in the sample). The researchers interviewed participants about any possible current symptoms, but importantly, when they struck upon anything that met criteria for a disorder, they also asked participants to *reflect back* to when they thought these symptoms first began. In this study, Kessler and colleagues found that, of all the participants who met criteria for a psychiatric disorder as adults, 75% of them reported first experiencing this disorder by the age of twenty-four, and 50% by the age of fourteen.

Neither study is perfect. The US study was much bigger – over 9,000 participants, compared to 1,000 in the NZ one. But the latter has a more reliable *prospective* design – events were tracked in real time, as they happened, rather than the US study's *retrospective* design, which relies on people's memory. The samples are also from within specific countries and cultures, so it's not clear if we can generalise these findings to other places. But the main take-home message is this: both studies agree that the majority of mental illness begins by the age of twenty-four. If you make it to the age of twenty-five without experiencing a mental illness, the chances that you'll get one beyond that age – while it certainly does happen – are reduced considerably.

When is adolescence?

Broadly, adolescence is defined as the period of physical and psychological development between childhood and adulthood, but determining the exact ages at which it begins and ends is trickier. For each individual, adolescence officially starts at the onset of puberty, when levels of hormones in the body start to increase rapidly (particularly oestrogen in girls, and testosterone in boys). It's hard to make a sweeping claim about when this happens though. The average age of puberty onset for girls is eleven and boys is twelve, but there is a lot of variation.[3] Organisations like the WHO state that adolescence starts with the second decade of life, at age ten, and that's a useful approximation for us to use here.[4]

It's also tricky to work out the average age at which adolescence ends. Legally, you become an adult when you turn eighteen. But how many of us truly feel or behave like 'an adult' on our eighteenth birthday? If you think adolescence lasts beyond eighteen, you're in good company. Many researchers argue that adolescence extends way beyond this point, for both biological and societal reasons. About twenty-five years ago, the prevailing knowledge was that brain development ended in childhood. Then those noisy, doughnut-shaped, room-sized brain scanners called magnetic resonance imaging (MRI) machines were developed. These gave researchers access to unprecedented detail about the brain, in terms of its structure (the size of different regions and how densely the cells in them are packed), its function (the activity within those regions), and its connectivity (how different regions communicate with each other). Evidence from MRI studies showed that the brain continues to change in all these dimensions well into the twenties, and in some cases, beyond that. Your brain has definitely not reached full maturity by your eighteenth birthday. This means that many of the things you do, feel and think – psychological processes that are underpinned by your brain – haven't reached full maturity either. Sarah-Jayne Blakemore, a cognitive neuroscientist who studies adolescence, says, 'Teenagers often *look* like adults – they are in adult bodies – but their brains are not adult at all.'[5]

There are societal factors to consider too. For most people in Western societies, few of the traditional markers of adulthood, like being financially independent from parents, getting married and having babies, apply at the age of eighteen. In fact, in the twenty-first century, these markers are being pushed further and further back, well into the twenties and thirties. In 1945, the average age of first marriage was 24.6 for men and 22.3 for women; in 2016 (for opposite-sex couples) it was 33.4 for men and 31.5 for women.[6] If adulthood doesn't really begin until the mid-twenties and thirties, then by definition adolescence hasn't ended by then either. Of course, everyone is different, and these markers are imperfect (a person in her thirties who lives with her parents because she can't afford to move out, for example, is not still an adolescent). But averages are useful. Taking all this into account – puberty, brain development, societal norms, the imperfect nature of making generalisations – researchers have suggested that the average end point of adolescence is twenty-four years.[7] So a reasonable age range for adolescence is something like ten to twenty-four years old.

In my experience, the idea that adolescence lasts this long comes as good news to people in their late teens and early twenties. As a lecturer, I taught a module on adolescent social development, and when I asked undergraduate students – largely eighteen-to-twenty-one-year-olds – what they thought about adolescence continuing until the age of twenty-four, they usually said they were relieved. Knowing they're still changing helps them feel better about various aspects of their life, like their mood or the choices they've made.

Why mental illness (often) starts in adolescence

In the previous chapter, we concluded that mental illness occurs because some people have an underlying vulnerability – biological and psychological – that is then 'triggered', either by something internal and biological or by an external source of stress. Broadly, adolescence is a period of risk for mental illness because it's one long series of these potential triggers. A pre-existing genetic vulnerability that lies dormant in childhood can come 'online' in adolescence, either triggered by the biological changes inherent to this age period, the stressful events that happen at this time, or both.

It helps to understand what this time of life – when it goes smoothly – is actually for. Put simply: the whole goal of adolescence is to develop from a vulnerable, dependent child into a mature, independent adult capable of sexual reproduction. If all goes well, adolescence involves a series of changes that gradually allow a person to support and look after themselves, manage complex social interactions, and navigate sexual relationships. But it's this exact series of changes that can, for some people, trigger a mental disorder.

Pubertal hormones activate two key processes required for the transition to adulthood. First, hormones help the body *physically* develop, to become a body that wants and is able to have sex and, for females, that can carry a child. Second, there must be psychological development. There are a host of cognitive and emotional skills needed to become a fully independent adult, capable of things that children cannot do, or at least not at a sufficiently mature level. Adults reflect on their past behaviour, plan for the future, evaluate information to make complex decisions, resist temptation, and consider the thoughts and feelings of others. (Of course, we can all think of adults who don't do these things particularly well ... but the idea, at least, is that adults are generally better at these tasks than children.) It's these processes – the bodily and psychological changes – that are developing so fundamentally in adolescence, and that will help us understand mental illness at this age.

The likelihood of an adolescent having a mental illness is linked to what stage of puberty they're in (i.e. their 'pubertal status'). Across many mental illnesses, there is a sharp rise in rates of mental disorders specifically once a young person hits puberty, including depression, anxiety disorders, conduct disorder and eating disorders. For example, one US study looked at the frequency of panic attacks in a group of eleven-to-thirteen-year-old girls.[8] Importantly, in this age range, some girls haven't started puberty, some are in its late stages, and others fall somewhere in between. The researchers found that all the girls who had experienced a panic attack (8% of the sample) were in the later stages of puberty; none of them were prepubertal or in the early stages. The same pattern is seen for many other disorders and their symptoms. This tells us that there is something specific about pubertal hormones – and not just being of a certain age – that is increasing the risk of these problems.

Changes to the body in adolescence

Let's first consider how the *physical* changes caused by puberty might increase a person's risk of mental illness by examining eating disorders in adolescent girls. (The majority of research into adolescent eating disorders has been conducted in girls.) A person with an eating disorder has a highly dysfunctional relationship with food. The two most well-known eating disorders are anorexia nervosa, characterised by extreme low weight, a fear of being fat, and restrictive eating; and bulimia nervosa, characterised by a pattern of binge eating and purging (either by vomiting, extreme exercise or use of laxatives). However, like most mental illnesses, disordered eating doesn't always fall neatly into one of these categories and, as mentioned earlier, some people binge without purging, so there is the additional diagnosis of binge-eating disorder. In addition, many symptoms are shared between anorexia and bulimia: binging and/or purging can appear in anorexia; people with bulimia show an extreme preoccupation with their weight. To get around this, the DSM-5 distinguishes the two disorders primarily by the person's weight – people with anorexia are severely underweight; people with bulimia are not.

Sadly, having a somewhat unhealthy relationship with food and your body is extremely common in adolescent girls, and indeed adult women. There have been strides towards improving the diversity of body shapes that are deemed acceptable in our culture, but we still have a long way to go. This was summed up nicely by the writer Jia Tolentino, who said that we are still preoccupied with the idea that girls and women need to be beautiful at all:

Mainstream feminism has also driven the movement toward what's called 'body acceptance', which is the practice of valuing women's beauty at every size and in every iteration ... These changes are overdue and positive, but they are double-edged. The default assumption [still] tends to be that it is politically

important to designate everyone as beautiful, that it is a meaningful project to make sure that everyone can become, and feel,
increasingly beautiful. We have hardly tried to imagine what
it might look like if our culture could do the opposite – de-
escalate the situation, make beauty matter *less*.[9]

But until all of that changes (I'm not holding my breath),
we remain in a culture where beauty and thinness are deemed
important, and by extension, a culture where unhealthy relationships with food and our bodies are common. But like
everything else dysfunctional, these symptoms lie on a spectrum,
and it is the extreme end of that spectrum – the eating-disorders
end – that we are focusing on now.

It is well established that puberty is a risk factor for eating
disorders: the vast majority of girls who develop an eating
disorder have already started puberty.[10] Consider what happens to girls' bodies during this time. Their breasts develop
and they put on weight, they grow body hair, they may experience skin problems like acne. This happens at an unfortunate
time: the exact time that brain development and increased
time with peers means adolescents care more about what
people think of them (more on that later). This can then
kick off a problematic chain of feelings and behaviours. If a
teenage girl thinks her classmates are judging her appearance
negatively – she's too overweight, her skin is too spotty, her
breasts are too small, whatever it might be – then she can
start to feel self-conscious and start to dislike her body. She
might have imagined these criticisms and judgements, or they
might have been explicitly said. Either way, she might then
try and lose weight to change her appearance, and turn to
dieting and/or exercise to achieve this. This can lead to a
restrictive relationship with food, in which calories are closely
monitored or certain foods are banned, and to obsessive
exercising (spending hours at the gym, trying to burn off all
calories consumed).

As I've said, these leanings are fairly common – sadly – in adolescent girls and women. But notice that these thoughts, feelings and behaviours are also symptoms of eating disorders, the ones just described. If these processes start to balloon or to take over a girl's life, an eating disorder can develop. Therefore, one way that puberty can contribute to an eating disorder is because it triggers changes in physical appearance. This isn't the only route by which an eating disorder develops, and there are many other factors at play, but this serves to illustrate how bodily changes – at least in part – can influence development of a disorder.

The *timing* of puberty is also important. All girls are at an elevated risk of developing an eating disorder once they start puberty, but for girls who start the process earlier than their friends, the risk is higher still.[11] (Eating disorders are still rare, of course; we are talking about relative risk here.) In fact, this phenomenon is true for many psychological and behavioural problems. For girls, beginning puberty early is also associated with an increased risk of depression, panic attacks, antisocial behaviour and substance abuse. But when it comes to eating disorders, starting puberty early can magnify the process I've described above. Early developers must navigate these potentially daunting body changes – periods, body odour, acne – on their own, under the glare of very young classmates who haven't yet been there themselves and don't understand. This can take its toll. Girls who start puberty early are more likely to report being unhappy with their bodies than those who start later, and more likely to have low self-esteem – both of which are risk factors for eating disorders. There is some evidence that this poor body image can persist in these girls, even once their friends have caught up and started puberty themselves.[12]

Importantly though, these risk factors (a changing body, judgement from peers, early puberty) don't set off a mental illness in *everyone*. We need to remember: these events will be a trigger for *some* girls, those who already had an underlying genetic and/or environmental vulnerability to developing psychiatric problems. For everyone else, these experiences will just be part of the sometimes awkward and uncomfortable process of growing up.

As an aside: the role of pubertal timing in boys' mental health problems is less clear. It was initially thought that starting puberty early could actually be an *advantage* for boys: the increased height, muscle mass and deep voice could confer some protective social status amongst classmates, which in theory could reduce the risk of social or emotional problems. However, exact findings are mixed, with some studies finding that both early and late puberty can be a risk factor for mental health problems in boys, and others finding no relationship between boys' pubertal timing and mental health.[13]

Changes to psychology in adolescence

With eating disorders, there's a clear link between changes in the body and an increased risk of mental illness. But there are lots of disorders which appear in adolescence – most of them, in fact – that haven't anything to do with bodily development or how we feel about our appearance. Pubertal hormones must also be doing something else. Indeed, even with eating disorders – where the physical body has such obvious significance – the risk of puberty derives from far more than the bodily changes taking place. A host of psychological changes also take place in puberty – the cognitive and emotional developments that are needed to prepare a young person for independent adult life.

Pubertal hormones trigger significant changes across the brain, both in terms of anatomical structure, levels of brain activity, and connections between regions. This continues right through the teenage years and beyond. And the brain, of course, is the route through which we experience all our psychology. Unsurprisingly, then, pretty much all our psychological faculties undergo significant development in adolescence, but the processes that are most pertinent for our purposes and that I'm going to focus on particularly relate to *social* interactions. This is partly because a full description of adolescent psychological development could fill a whole book but also because so much of adolescence – and mental illness at this age – ultimately comes back to social development.

To become independent, find emotional support beyond the family, and find and keep a sexual partner, an adolescent must develop nuanced, sophisticated social skills. A lot of the psychological changes happening in adolescents are therefore related to how we perceive, respond to, think about and interact with other people. For this reason, adolescence is known as a period of significant 'social reorientation', during which relationships with peers take centre stage and becoming increasingly sophisticated and complex.[14]

In order to achieve social competence, we must develop a key capacity: the ability to understand what other people are thinking and feeling. Every time we speak to someone else, we need to be able to understand their meaning but also to read between the lines of what they are saying to grasp the subtext; we need to identify sarcasm and jokes and lies. We must interpret a person's tone of voice, facial expressions and body language. We need to figure out who agrees with us, who is criticising us, who is flirting with us, often from brief exchanges. This multifaceted ability to identify other people's mental states, so fundamental to all our social interactions, is known as 'theory of mind' or 'mentalising'. (It is this particular skill that is often limited or dysfunctional in individuals with autism spectrum disorder, which can lead to problems with social interactions and relationships.) In typically developing individuals, theory of mind becomes increasingly complex and sophisticated across the adolescent years. But this necessary shifting of focus onto other people's minds and behaviour – particularly that of peers – can lead to a lot of problems too.

Our self-concept – the image we have of ourselves, the collection of traits and stories that we feel make us unique – is developing rapidly in adolescence. Children's self-concept tends to be quite concrete and straightforward: they think and describe themselves in terms of their age, their name, their likes and dislikes. In adolescence, the self-concept rapidly becomes more abstract and complex. People view themselves in terms of their personality, values and beliefs.[15] As Sarah-Jayne Blakemore says: 'During adolescence, your sense of who you are – your moral and political beliefs, your music and fashion tastes, what social group you associate with – undergoes profound change. During adolescence, we are inventing ourselves.'[16]

Critically, adolescents also start incorporating what *other people* think about them into their sense of self. Because children's ability to represent others' minds is more rudimentary, other people's attitudes and feelings don't feature so prominently in their self-concept. But in adolescence, when we become better able to understand what other people think about us, their opinions become richly interwoven into our understanding of who we are.

If an adolescent is popular and has warm and supportive friendships and relationships, this is not a problem. But if an adolescent is treated badly by those around them, it can affect their fundamental sense of self. As noted in the previous chapter, if they are mocked or insulted or ignored by their peers, they can believe it's because they are uncool or worthless. This is dangerous because a healthy, positive view of ourselves is critical in protecting ourselves against mental illness. As will be familiar by now, many people with eating disorders or depression, for example, dislike or hate themselves or their body, and feel that they have low worth or are unlovable. Equally, an adolescent could have close friendships but still *believe* that others are judging them extremely negatively, as happens in social anxiety disorder, again leading to negative beliefs about themselves. In fact, social anxiety disorder has been referred to as the 'prototypical adolescent disorder'[17] because it represents so clearly what can happen when a fundamental process of adolescence, the 'social reorientation', goes awry. Either way, adolescents' acute concern about what others think about them can make some individuals vulnerable to mental disorder.

Related to this is the concept of social exclusion or rejection. In 2010, a group of researchers led by Catherine Sebastian studied the effects of social exclusion on mood and anxiety levels.[18] To do this, they used a computer game called Cyberball, in which the participant plays a simple game of catch with two cartoon characters on screen. The participant is told that the characters are being controlled by other real participants, in a different room or school, when in fact the pattern of throwing and catching is preprogrammed by the computer. There are two rounds: first, the characters include the participant in the game, throwing the ball back and forth to her. But in the second round, they initially pass the ball to the participant, but then start to ignore her, passing the ball only between themselves. Sebastian and colleagues asked three age groups to play this game: what they called young adolescents (11.9–13.9 years old), mid-adolescents (14–15.8 years old) and adults (22.2–47.1 years old).

All participants reported feeling more ignored and excluded after the second round of the game. (In fact, the effect is very powerful: other studies have shown that people feel rejected even when they know the characters are controlled by a computer.[19]) But, based on questionnaires given throughout the experiment, the *emotional* impact of being excluded was greater for the younger participants. For both adolescent groups (but not the adults), mood levels dropped significantly after the second game. For the youngest group only, anxiety levels significantly increased. This effect was very fleeting – the intention was not to cause harm to the participants – but the experiment perfectly captures the fact that feeling left out has a bigger impact in your teenage years.

This has since been supported by several other studies. The hypothesis is that it hurts more because fitting in with peers is so deeply important in adolescence, but also because, at that age, we are less good at regulating our emotional reactions to upsetting events, something we get better at as we mature.[20]

In adolescence we also develop our capacity to experience *social emotions*, a term psychologists use to refer to emotions that are specifically dependent on other people, such as guilt and shame. If we weren't aware of, or didn't care about, how our actions affected other people or what they thought about us, we'd never experience these emotions. They exist to some extent in childhood, but it's in adolescence – when we are suddenly so interested in what others think and feel about us – that they ramp up.[21] Again, experiencing sensible levels of these emotions is important: the personality disorder psychopathy tells us what can happen to social behaviour when someone experiences very little guilt or shame. But these emotions become a problem when we feel them too readily or too extensively. Excessive levels of guilt and shame are a common feature of many mental disorders, including depression and anxiety disorders. Again, it's easy to see how an essential adolescent process – caring about how our actions affect others – can send some people on the path to mental illness.

There is one more social process that is ramping up in adolescence: paranoia. When someone worries excessively that others are hostile towards them or out to harm them, we describe them as paranoid. When a paranoid belief is extreme, held tightly in the face of all counter-evidence, and very disruptive to a person's life, it becomes a paranoid *delusion*, and this is a symptom of psychotic disorders like schizophrenia. Paranoia in children is rare. Instead, our tendency to feel paranoid develops in adolescence, peaking in the early twenties.[22] Again, this is useful for navigating new relationships with our peers – for detecting who to apologise to, for example, or who is a threat. But it's this exact skill that, when it goes off the rails, can lead to a risk of (particularly psychotic) mental disorders at this age.

In summary, adolescence is partly a period of risk because it is a period of social reorientation. A great deal of the biological and psychological changes in adolescence make a young person think and care about other people their age: friends, classmates, romantic partners and strangers. Adolescents care deeply about who likes them, whether their actions and tastes and appearance are accepted by their peers, and what their social standing is. All of this sets them up well for adulthood. But it's also their acute sensitivity to these things that can make some of them vulnerable to mental illness.

What's happening in the outside world?

The biological and psychological changes of adolescence don't occur in a vacuum. Adolescents are also contending with an external social world, one that's very different to what they experienced in childhood, and that's really important for understanding the onset of mental illness too. Something significant happens in the outside world around the start of adolescence: children move to secondary school or high school.

Around the start of secondary school, the responsibility for planning a young person's social life starts to shift, from parents to the young person themselves. Parent-sanctioned playdates are replaced by adolescent-driven, unsupervised socialising. This is facilitated by mobile phones: many young people get their first phone around the start of secondary school, enabling more independent planning. This is all significant not just because it means more time spent with peers away from parents, but because they are a *new* set of peers. The cosy familiarity of primary-school classmates – who in many cases have remained a consistent group since the age of four or five – is suddenly replaced with a huge new pool of potential friends, enemies and rivals. Alongside their new-found independence, young adolescents are also navigating a new social hierarchy – the very concept of which barely existed to them before – and trying to figure out where their place in it might be.

Meanwhile, thanks to puberty, adolescents start to become sexually attracted to their peers. With the commencement of secondary school, adolescents can suddenly find themselves spending an awful lot of unsupervised time cooped up with the very peers that they're biologically most interested in. Assuming the young person can find someone who reciprocates their attraction (not always an easy task), the new levels of independence – the private communication via phones, the lack of parental supervision – means it's now actually possible to have sexual relationships. (In the academic literature, a person's first experience of sex is referred to as their 'sexual debut', which I rather like, as to me it conjures up images of feather boas and jazz hands.) Maybe this goes reasonably smoothly: two teenagers are in a committed, trusting relationship; the sexual activity is consensual and private; the relationship ends mutually and maturely. But it rarely works out like this.

Sex can also trigger all kinds of potential stress. It might cause friction or arguments between friends; rumours might be spread; people might be pressured into having sex; there could be unwanted pregnancies or STIs. Compromising photos could get into the wrong hands: many 'sexts' are sent between teenagers without incident, but when intimate photos are shared widely across a school, for example, the psychological consequences can be severe. Even if the sex itself doesn't cause difficulties, relationship problems like being cheated on or being dumped can be humiliating or heartbreaking. In short, two key features of adolescence – biological interest in sex and a new, independent social life – can lead to the kind of stressful life events that sometimes spark off a mental illness.

The sheer fact that adolescents are out and about more, away from their parents, spending more time in the world, can also increase their risk of events that might lead to mental illness, such as an assault or car crash leading to PTSD or a frightening event leading to an anxiety disorder. The tendency to take risks, and the desire for extreme physical and psychological experiences ('sensation seeking'), both peak in adolescence. This is partly why adolescents may want to take drugs or binge drink – and adolescence is also usually the first time these substances become available to them. Equally, being especially anxious about what others think of them, some adolescents may feel pressured into taking risks, including drinking and taking drugs, in order to fit in. Drinking and drug-taking tend to peak in late adolescence and early adulthood, and then decline after that. Of course, most teenagers (and adults) experiment in this way without any particularly negative consequences, but for a minority these behaviours introduce or reveal a susceptibility to mental illness that didn't exist or wasn't apparent in childhood. Substance use can lead to mental disorder directly via addiction, or because it triggers symptoms of other disorders, such as cannabis causing anxiety and paranoia. And of course being under the influence further increases the likelihood of encountering risky situations where traumas like car accidents or assault can occur.

Sleep: adding fuel to the fire

Finally, another biological process that changes dramatically in adolescence and is intimately linked with mental illness is sleep. For a host of biological and social reasons, adolescents generally don't feel sleepy until later at night and need to sleep for longer in the mornings.[23] While some people are naturally early birds and others are night owls, in adolescence everyone shifts a bit towards the night-owl end of the spectrum. This means that many adolescents are operating with a chronic sleep deficit: for some young people who can't fall asleep until very late, waking up for school is like getting up in the middle of the night.

In part to compensate for this, and in part because of late-night socialising, adolescents often have a very different sleeping pattern at weekends compared to in the week, sleeping well into late morning or the afternoon. This contrast between weekday and weekend sleeping habits leads to a phenomenon called 'social jetlag', where yo-yoing between the two sleep schedules is similar to constantly jumping between time zones.[24] All of this was the case even before mobile phones were added into the mix: devices that tempt adolescents to stay up even later to continue playing games or socialising with their friends.[25] In short, adolescents often have chronically disrupted, suboptimal sleep.

This is highly relevant because sleep problems can cause or exacerbate the very processes that lead to mental illness. Even short-term lack of sleep makes it harder to regulate your emotions, for example.[26] This is true for everyone, not just adolescents, but in adolescence emotion regulation is quite poor anyway and is particularly poor for those who develop a mental illness. It's easy to slip into a cycle in which sleep problems exacerbate symptoms and then symptoms (particularly rumination and anxiety) make it harder to sleep. In this way, sleep can be yet another trigger – something that is changing anyway in adolescence but can set off mental illness in some individuals.

For vulnerable individuals, adolescence is a time of great risk for all of the reasons touched on in this chapter. In this minority of adolescents, the complex physical and psychological development necessary for becoming an independent adult can go awry – in the words of neuroscientist Jay Giedd and colleagues, 'anomalies or exaggerations of typical adolescent maturation processes' put them on a path to potential mental illness.[27] But it's important to remember that they are only a minority. Adolescence can be a bumpy ride, but most people get through it unscathed. As I will explain later in the book, this is why I think we need to be really careful about the messages we give parents, teachers and young people about mental health. Lots of adolescents have periods of being down or anxious or moody, and that's not any particular cause for concern, certainly not medical concern. Adolescence involves periods of stress, and we need to learn how to navigate that without feeling there is something abnormal going on, or that a doctor or therapist needs to be called.

One last subject remains before we address the question of why rates of mental illness might be increasing today. I've deliberately avoided much mention of the topic in this chapter because I want to make clear that there's so much else happening in adolescence. But we're going to turn to this topic now because it is, without question, a central part of adolescents' (and adults') lives and is often the first suspect to be accused of causing mental distress and disorder. So: what impact does social media really have on mental health?

CHAPTER 7

Social media

According to many headlines and informal conversations, social media is having a devastating effect on people's mental health, particularly young people. In February 2019, for example, the *i* newspaper published an article with the headline 'Suicide rate almost doubles among teenagers, as social media giants are told they have a "duty of care" to tackle it'.[1] A few months later, during a roundtable discussion on children's mental health, Prince Harry said, 'Social media is more addictive than drugs and alcohol, yet it's more dangerous because it's normalised and there are no restrictions to it'.[2] He wasn't just saying it was equivalent to these substances, he was saying it was worse. In August 2019, several celebrities, including the models Gigi Hadid and Kaia Gerber, posted selfies showing the same phone case: one that read, in the style of a warning on a cigarette packet, 'Social media seriously harms your mental health'. (They posted the photos on ... yep, social media.)

This attitude is widespread. Intuitively, it feels right: in a relatively short space of time, we have transformed the way we communicate. Many of us spend hours on a device that's specifically designed to lock in our attention. This hasn't just affected young people, but most of the discussion, and concern, is that this shift in behaviour is having a seriously harmful effect on their well-being. A lot of the time, it isn't even up for debate; we talk about the psychological cost of social media like it's a universal fact. But the truth is rather more complicated.

Conflicting findings

In 2018, a landmark paper came out from the States, with more than 500,000 participants aged between thirteen and eighteen.[3] This study found that digital screen use (any screen use besides schoolwork) and depressive symptoms were linked: across the sample, both girls and boys who clocked up more hours of screen time had higher scores on a depression questionnaire. For girls only, there was also a positive correlation between hours spent on social media specifically and depressive symptoms. The lead author, Jean Twenge, wrote up the findings in a book called *iGen*, an adaptation of which was published as an article in *The Atlantic* – 'Have smartphones destroyed a generation?' – which has been shared nearly 800,000 times online. In the article, she writes: 'The twin rise of the smartphone and social media has caused an earthquake of a magnitude we've not seen in a very long time, if ever. There is compelling evidence that the devices we've placed in young people's hands are having profound effects on their lives – and making them seriously unhappy.'[4]

For many, this was job done: scientific confirmation of what they already knew. But the academic community – other researchers studying adolescence or mental health or tech use – were up in arms about this article, particularly the wording that Twenge used.

The first problem they identified with the study was that, as with lots of research on social media, the information about both phone usage and mental health symptoms were collected at a single point in time (making it a cross-sectional, rather than longitudinal, study). If you find a positive correlation between time spent on social media and depressive symptoms at one time point, you have no idea whether social media is *causing* the depressive symptoms, even though this is the conclusion that the authors presented. It could be, for example, that people who are already depressed are the ones who tend to go on social media more: maybe they've withdrawn from their friends, so they spend more time on their phone; maybe they find it comforting or easier to connect to people online when feeling down. Or it could be that a third variable – lack of sleep, for example – is causing both the increase in social media use and the increase in depressive symptoms. If an adolescent has insomnia, this could mean they go on their phone more (because they are literally awake for longer) and it could also mean they are more likely to be depressed (insomnia increases your risk for developing depression). From a cross-sectional correlation alone, we just have no idea which of these options is correct. But the language used by these researchers, and the Twenge book based on the study, argued that social media use led to depression. This is obviously poor scientific practice, but with this topic it's socially irresponsible too: creating alarm and panic (and parental rules) before we have all the facts.

The authors were also criticised for the flawed statistical approach they took, because it increased the size of the relationship between social media and depression, and also increased the likelihood that the relationship was found at all. A later study based in the UK, led by Amy Orben at the University of Oxford, used a more robust statistical approach.[5] This study used data from 12,000 ten-to-fifteen-year-olds, taken from a large, nationally representative database. This one was a longitudinal study – the researchers had data from eight time points, between 2009 and 2016 – which meant it was possible to look at relationships between variables across time. The researchers measured two things: the number of hours the young person spent on social media each day, and how satisfied they reported feeling with their life. (Low life satisfaction is not, of course, a measure of mental illness but is widely regarded as a useful proxy for mental health problems.)

The results suggested little cause for alarm. They did find a negative relationship between social media use and life satisfaction, in both directions (increased social media use was related to later decreased life satisfaction, and decreased life satisfaction was related to later increased social media use), and that this relationship was slightly stronger in girls. But importantly, the size of this relationship was tiny. They found that 99.6% of the variation in girls' life satisfaction had nothing to do with their social media use. In other words, if I knew how many hours an adolescent was spending on social media each day, this information would allow me to accurately predict just 0.4% of her total life satisfaction score. The rest would be down to other factors, like her health, her family's finances and whether or not she was being bullied, for example. To put it in Orben's words: 'These effects were minuscule by the standards of science and trivial if you want to inform personal parenting decisions.'[6]

Another longitudinal study specifically assessed anxiety and depression symptoms (rather than life satisfaction) over eight years – although the sample was much smaller (500 thirteen-to-twenty-year-olds).[7] This 2020 study, led by Sarah Coyne in the US, found no relationship in either direction: when an adolescent spent more time on social media relative to their own average use, they didn't experience a subsequent increase in anxiety or depression; nor did they experience a drop in these symptoms when they started using social media less.

This all feels reassuring: based on robust, longitudinal studies, hours spent on social media don't seem to be linked to increased mental health symptoms. But it doesn't give us the full story. Anyone who uses these apps knows that an hour on social media can mean a lot of different things; social media use is not a single behaviour. There are a lot of different apps, for starters, which have different features – some are more about looking at videos, for example; some are more about messaging people. Even within the same app, there are different ways to spend your time. On Instagram, you can spend an hour editing pictures of yourself, or you can spend an hour watching funny videos from celebrities, or you can have a one-to-one chat with a friend (amongst other things). What we actually *do* on social media varies a lot: from person to person, and even within the same person, depending on the day. If we want to understand how social media affects mental health, then surely we need to look in a bit more detail at *how* people are spending their time on the apps, rather than simply measuring the number of hours they are on them. We need to think about specific social media behaviours and the underlying psychological processes they tap into, and what these might mean for mental health.

When the self-concept goes online

A good place to start is the question of how social media might affect and interact with a person's self-concept, as we know this to be developing rapidly in adolescence and a critical factor in several mental disorders. One common social media behaviour is that people broadcast information about themselves and their lives in the form of photos, written statements and videos – some that exist only fleetingly, others that can be viewed and shared endlessly. Importantly, this involves making choices about what they post and how to present themselves. This kind of 'impression management' exists offline as well, of course. To manage other people's views of us, we are continually choosing which stories to tell about ourselves, controlling our behaviour, adjusting how we look with make-up, haircuts or certain clothes. We do this, consciously or unconsciously, to present a particular version of ourselves to other people – a flattering one. In 'real life', though, we are broadcasting ourselves live, all the time, so inevitably some less favourable facial expressions or hair days or behaviours will slip through. Online, we can withhold or delete anything that doesn't suit the exact message we want to send about ourselves. The extent to which our self-image can be controlled on social media takes impression management to a whole new level, and there's long been a concern that curating your image like this might be psychologically harmful.

There's some tentative evidence to support this. One 2020 study looked at the posting of selfies in a group of fourteen-to-seventeen-year-old girls in the US.[8] The researchers found that participants who were more 'invested' in selfies, and spent more time editing them, were more likely to score highly on a measure of *self-objectification* – the tendency to view your own worth as dependent on your body and appearance. This in turn was associated with more anxiety and shame about their appearance. However, this study was cross-sectional, not longitudinal, so it tells us nothing about whether selfie-editing causes people to dislike their bodies or whether people who have a more fragile relationship with their body are more likely to spend time and effort editing their selfies.

A study in 2018 investigated this question of causality – specifically, whether posting selfies might make people more anxious about their appearance.[9] In this case, researchers asked female undergraduate participants to complete questionnaires assessing their current level of anxiety and how they felt about their body, and then randomly split them into three groups. The first group were asked to take a single photo of themselves on the researcher's iPad and upload it to their own social media profile straight away. In the second group, participants were asked to take several photos of themselves, choose the one that they preferred, edit it using photo editing software (if they wished), and then upload it to their social media profile. The third group, which acted as a control, were asked to read a news article on the iPad. All groups then waited for a few minutes, before answering the same questionnaires from the start of the experiment. The researchers found that participants in the selfie groups reported feeling more anxious, less confident, and less physically attractive after the task, regardless of whether they had been able to choose and edit their photo, whereas the control group did not. This study provides an interesting clue – although the sample size was small – that broadcasting selfies may have at least a temporary negative effect on how people feel.

Receiving feedback

But posting information about ourselves is only half the story. On most apps, when we post something, we *receive feedback* on what we post, normally in the form of 'likes'. These tiny, instant, easy-tap hearts may be key to understanding some online behaviour, including the harm it can cause. Consider the words of one twenty-year-old writer, Ellie Pool: 'For me, if an Instagram post "flops", so doesn't get the normal amount of likes my posts average at, my confidence falls through the floor. The questions start running through my head: do I look fat in this picture? Do I look ugly in this picture? Does my face look weird? Do my legs look too big? Does my figure look chubby? And on, and on, and on.'[10]

In the offline world, we've always cared about signals that others like us: we notice whether they smile at us, compliment us, invite us to spend time together. But social media takes our age-old desire for social approval and changes it in two interesting and potentially harmful ways. First, it becomes quantifiable: it's possible, as the quote above shows, to track exactly how 'liked' your post is and how it compares to your average. Second, it's public: your approval rating is available for everyone else to see, potentially a wide audience. By the same token, you can also see the likes that other people have received. In real life, we've always wondered what others think of us, and wondered whether other people are more popular than we are. Online, there are clearly visible metrics that purport to answer these questions.

The fear is that likes are catnip, especially for young people, and that not getting enough of them drives unhealthy behaviour (such as obsessive checking) and makes people feel anxious and unhappy. Anecdotally, it's clear that adolescents place great value on this form of social approval. Some will delete posts that they feel haven't received enough likes, some use hashtags such as 'likeforlike', meaning they are willing to give a stranger an endorsement in exchange for one in return.

On the video-sharing app TikTok, adolescents are sometimes explicit about what they want when they post: 'Please don't let this flop.'

So there is some scientific evidence that posting selfies may have a negative effect on our feelings about ourselves, and there is plenty of anecdotal evidence that people care a great deal about how their posts are received because of the potential to quantify and compare their popularity. But before we start making any assumptions about the deleterious effect of this activity on mental health, it's important to remember what we know about the complex and multifactorial causes of mental illness. Crucially, we need to remember that none of this social media activity happens in a vacuum.

At the start of Pool's article quoted above, she writes: 'I have never been confident in my appearance. I have suffered with disordered eating, a lot of anxiety and insecurity about my appearance and going through a break-up which was fuelled by infidelity has only lowered my opinion of myself even further.' I don't mean to single her out. She is one of hundreds of thousands of teenagers and adults posting content about themselves online, and tracking the reaction it gets. My point is that everyone posting online has their own particular vulnerabilities, background and real-life social context that influence their relationship with social media in an important way. Some people sharing pictures of themselves will be predisposed to low self-worth, or disordered eating, or social anxiety through their combination of genetics and psychology and life experiences. And for *those* people, some aspects of social media – particularly the posting-and-getting-feedback bits – have the potential to be fraught and dysfunctional, sometimes seriously so. But that is distinctly different from the conclusion that 'social media seriously harms everyone's mental health'.

We don't yet have the data to draw any firm conclusions, but a more convincing argument, to my mind, is that broadcasting information and receiving feedback fuels a rich-get-richer, poor-get-poorer phenomenon. For confident people with lots of friends, social media likely serves as an amplifier of their stable self-confidence and popularity, their existing social status confirmed by a flood of online approval. For those who are insecure or lonely in the real world, social media is also an amplifier, but this time of the fragile self-esteem or uncertain social status they feel so intensely in real life. For this reason, we need to fine-tune our concerns about social media to focus on teenagers (and adults) who are *already vulnerable* to the kind of problems and processes that social media can exaggerate. For people with an underlying propensity for disordered eating, say, comparison with other people via social media, or online advice about dieting, could reasonably be the 'trigger' that tips them over into a full-blown eating disorder. But even then, we need to be cautious in our assessment of whether social media is creating a new problem or whether these people might have ended up unwell anyway, just with a different trigger. When it comes to sharing content about ourselves, social media may be a mirror that reflects and in some cases amplifies a person's existing life and difficulties, rather than a portal into a new world.

Viewing harmful content online

In November 2017, there was an awful case of a fourteen-year-old British girl, Molly Russell, taking her own life. After her death, her family discovered she had been looking at a great deal of content on social media relating to depression, self-harm and suicide. She hadn't told her family she was struggling. Her dad, Ian Russell, was quoted as saying that Instagram 'helped kill my daughter'.[11]

Since Molly's death, Instagram has vowed to remove images and drawings relating to self-harm and suicide. In November 2019, the platform reported that they had removed almost 1.7 million posts between April and September that year, over 9,000 a day. They also stated that only four in every 10,000 views involved such an image, although it's not clear what the statistic had been before their intervention.[12] But it remains a simple matter to find content online describing mental health problems or illness.

At the time of writing, a search on Tumblr for 'depression' leads to a screen reading 'Everything Okay?' followed by a series of links to mental illness advice helplines and the option to 'Go back'. Click on 'View search results', though, and an endlessly scrollable wall of posts appears. The majority of them are words superimposed onto images, often black and white. There are pictures of people staring out of bus windows, pictures of the sea, of stars in the night sky. Phrases include, 'I have more scars than friends' and 'I just feel empty inside all the fucking time'. Some explicitly mention suicide: 'I want something to kill me so I don't have to do it myself'. One post shows the words 'I just need a break from life' over a black and white gif of a deserted street at night, raindrops caught in the street lights. These easy-to-find posts represent the tip of what is available online. In terms of eating disorders, the Internet has spawned the troubling phenomenon of 'proana' (pro-anorexia) sites and posts. These provide and encourage posts relating to the eating disorder, such as images of people with very low weight or tips for how to eat as little as possible. Social media platforms have clocked these posts, and searches for proana terms like 'thinspiration' usually now come up empty, but people have found more subtle ways to post and tag this content online. A bit of committed digging – particularly beyond the most popular apps – reveals a dark underworld of much more graphic, explicit content relating to mental disorders: images of self-harm, discussion of suicide methods. There is no question that this stuff is out there, masses of it. The trickier question is figuring out exactly what effect it's having.

One possibility is that online material makes absolutely no difference to a person's state of mind, that what matters is what's happening in real life. The people who are not susceptible to these symptoms are not changed by viewing these posts (and probably aren't looking for them in the first place), and the ones who are looking at them were at risk anyway; the posts are irrelevant. In other words, a person's level of mental health symptoms – including self-harm and suicidal behaviour – is entirely determined by what is happening outside, not inside, their phone.

Another possibility is more concerning: that viewing these posts triggers or exacerbates new levels of distress and disorder. Or in the case of suicide and self-harm, that they normalise self-injurious behaviour as a way of coping with overwhelming emotions – such posts 'give people the idea' of self-harming: presenting a way of coping that they might have not considered before, or might have considered too taboo. Seeing these posts either activates something entirely new in an individual, creating a mental illness that would otherwise never have existed, or it exaggerates symptoms in those who are already unwell, or it translates mental distress into new harmful physical behaviour. The concern is therefore that seeing these posts could shift someone further along the continuum of mental ill health or make their existing distress more likely to be physically dangerous or life-threatening.

It's very difficult to test out these two possibilities, because all research options are unethical or impractical. To know for sure what impact these posts have, you could, in theory, recruit a group of people who use social media and a control group of people who don't, and track and compare mental health symptoms (including self-harm and suicidal behaviour) in the two groups. This would allow you to see whether being on social media generally (which will likely involve some exposure to mental illness content) is harmful. But this approach would be difficult, particularly with adolescents. It's now quite unusual for a young person to not be on social media, so even if you could find such a group, they would likely differ from the social media group in other important ways. Maybe they would have different family circumstances, or more financial hardship, or different real-life friendships. Even if you found that they had different levels of mental health symptoms, you couldn't be sure that it was the lack of social media that was causing the difference. The alternative would be to get a group of people who are all on social media and then control the content that they see, allowing some of them to see posts relating to mental illness, self-harm and suicide, and some of them not, and then compare their mental health over the following weeks or months. But that would never get ethical approval: you can't experimentally expose people to content that might be harmful.

So we can't definitively measure what effect these images are having. But evidence from qualitative studies – those that interview a small number of participants and analyse what they say in lots of detail – suggest we have reason to be concerned. A study published in 2017 asked twenty-one adolescents (aged between sixteen and twenty-four) from Wales with a history of self-harm to discuss the role they think the Internet might have played in the behaviour.[13] The participants described how the images that they saw sometimes triggered or encouraged their own self-harm, and that their behaviour escalated after they started to look at this content online. One nineteen-year-old participant said:

> I was in complete secrecy about my self-harm, but then I'd go home and I had all these people on the computer who I could talk to, who would support me, who didn't see self-harm as some weird thing that was a massive problem. They saw, you know, they saw it the same as making a cup of tea in the morning when you wake up, it was completely fine. But the problem with that was my cuts went from scratches to a lot deeper.

We also have reason to be concerned about the role the Internet and social media might play in suicide. A review of this topic published in 2012 highlighted several problems: the Internet has allowed people to search for information online related to methods, and it can give them access to the thoughts of other vulnerable people contemplating the same thing.[14]

There are also online suicide notes (posting the equivalent of a suicide note as a social media update), which may be triggering for other vulnerable individuals.

Across many disorders and difficulties, then, social media and the Internet more broadly provide access to like-minded individuals, which could plant ideas or encourage or normalise harmful behavior. But the point remains. How would these affected people have fared in the absence of social media? If we ask them, as in qualitative studies, we certainly get the impression that social media can exacerbate problematic behaviour and be subjectively experienced as harmful. And as we'll explore in Chapter 8, it's relevant that self-harm has increased in recent years as social media use has proliferated. But we can't know for sure. In every person, the seeds of their vulnerability will likely have been planted long before they first went online, and they will be exposed simultaneously to many risk factors offline too.

Might social media be good for mental health?

We're also missing half the story here. When we think about young people looking at online content relating to mental illness, we think about the harm it might be doing. But there's also a lot of positive content about mental illness on the Internet too. A great deal of online activity relating to self-harm, for example, is actually about access to social support.

A US study from 2006 categorised 3,219 messages posted mostly by females aged twelve to twenty on 400 message boards and forums focused on self-harm.[15] They found that the largest category (28.3% of posts) were those in which people provided each other with informal help and support to reduce self-harm. A paper published in 2016 reviewed twenty-seven studies conducted over the previous decade that each assessed the potential role of the Internet and social media on self-harm behaviour.[16] The authors identified three ways in which the Internet might make self-harm worse: by encouraging or normalising that behaviour, by triggering the urge to self-harm and, should they encounter stigmatising rather than normalising content, by making people who self-harm feel ashamed of their behaviour. But they also identified four potential benefits: the reduction of social isolation for people who are self-harming or wanting to self-harm; encouragement of recovery; the opportunity to disclose and discuss difficult emotions and feelings; and the ability of all of the above to reduce the urge to self-harm. The title of their paper points to the contradiction the authors had identified: 'A double-edged sword: a review of benefits and risks of online non-suicidal self-injury activities'.

This phrase – a double-edged sword – could be used to summarise the relationship of social media with mental health as a whole. Alongside proana content, for example, there is also a lot of online material that supports recovery from eating disorders. One study that analysed eating-disorder content on Tumblr found there were more posts encouraging recovery and criticising the proana movement (63.2% of all content about eating disorders) than there were proana posts.[17] The Internet can provide suicidal people with access to methods and like-minded individuals, but it also presents many opportunities for suicide prevention. Charitable campaigns to promote awareness about suicide – such as how to speak to someone suicidal – are shared widely. Attempts to search for content about suicide on social media are now met with advice about how to get help, and phone lines to call. When in the past someone might have felt entirely alone, the Internet allows them to connect with others and find support. In summary, social media doesn't play a single role in any mental illness or mental health problem. It depends who you are, what you're looking for, and what you find.

Friends online

While social media certainly has a dark side – at times, a horribly dark side – social media can also be good for mental health for a very simple but often overlooked reason: because of the opportunity it offers for communication and connection. A review paper in 2018 posed the question: do the fundamental aspects of offline adolescent friendship also exist online?[18] The authors highlighted four aspects of real-life friendship. First, *validation*: friends confirm each other's self-worth by giving attention and compliments and making each other feel valued. Second, *self-disclosure*: friends share details about their lives. (In fact, it can be an interesting step to notice in the early stages of any new relationship, at any age – the moment when you decide to share something a little more personal about yourself.) Third, friends provide *instrumental support*, offering each other help and guidance. The fourth component is *companionship*: the entertainment aspect of friendship, the fact that friends have fun with one another.

The researchers found that all four components of adolescent friendship can be seen online. Of course, as we've already discussed, validation is rife on social media, in the form of likes but also complimentary comments on posts, or even simply receiving a reply to a WhatsApp message. Friends also regularly self-disclose to each other online, particularly in private messaging apps, sharing everything from the mundane to the monumental. One study found that adolescents go online to discuss the things that are stressing them out – and report feeling better for doing so;[19] another found that some adolescents find online disclosure easier and more helpful than talking about their feelings and experiences face to face.[20]

Adolescents also provide each other with instrumental support online: they contact each other via social media for homework help, for example, or for advice about outfits when shopping or getting ready to go out. Finally, there is a wealth of evidence that companionship exists on social media – that adolescents have fun with each other online. Friends share funny gifs and memes, make videos with each other dancing or messing around, and play video games together. For some reason I've never quite understood, this entertainment aspect of social media is almost entirely left out of the public conversation. Some social media apps can be an endless source of potential entertainment and comedy to share with your friends, for adults as well as teenagers. There is so much discussion about how these apps are designed to be 'addictive', to lure us with their devious tricks, but I think a key reason for their popularity might be far less sinister: it's a way of having fun with our friends.

Of course, social media giants have not created these apps out of the goodness of their hearts. Our enjoyment of them is partly because it gives us access to social connection, but this is a by-product of their design rather than their primary goal. We also return to these apps time and time again because they are cleverly designed to hook in our attention. For example, the system of likes draws on a classic psychological phenomenon known as *intermittent reinforcement*: rewards that are unpredictable give us the biggest kick. We know this from subjective reports – part of the fun of, for example, playing the lottery derives from our having no idea whether we will win or not – but also from brain-scanning studies that show the brain responds more when rewards are unpredictable.[21] This is exactly what is happening each time someone posts some content on social media – it might get a handful of likes, none at all, or a huge response – and with direct messaging (particularly, say, in the early stages of dating): if you're not sure if and when you'll get a response, or what the other person will say, then it feels better when it pays off. Another key feature of social media feeds is that they allow us to scroll almost indefinitely, not to mention that the content is tailored to our interests based on the store of data being gathered about our preferences.

But just because social media is designed to hold our attention in these various ways doesn't mean it can't be a powerful source of entertainment and social connection *at the same time*. It's a new manifestation of something we have always needed and wanted and enjoyed: to comfort, support and entertain each other.

The ugly side of online communication

If social media is a mirror reflecting the best of human relationships, it can also show us the worst. Because of course, in the real world, humans can be hideous and awful to each other, and that happens online too. We have touched on the ways that social media provides additional opportunities for bullying in adolescence – people can take humiliating photos and videos and share these online, for example – and the list of other ways people can be cruel to one another online will be sadly familiar: trolling with aggressive or insulting messages, impersonation, revenge porn, blackmail, and rape and death threats. Entirely unsurprisingly, being the target of this abuse can take its toll on mental health and, at its worst, it may increase risk of suicide. A 2014 meta-analysis of forty-three studies and over 300,000 participants found that being cyberbullied is associated with increased suicidal thoughts (although note that the studies were cross-sectional).[22]

What remains an open question is whether being bullied or abused online has a more negative effect on victims than the equivalent offline behaviours. An important point to consider is that the vast majority of young people who are bullied online are *also* being bullied in the real world. One 2017 study of over 2,700 UK adolescents found that just 1% of cyberbullying victims were 'only' being bullied online.[23] The authors, led by Dieter Wolke, concluded: 'Cyberbullying creates few new victims, but is mainly a new tool to harm victims already bullied by traditional means.' Nonetheless, there are certainly some reasons why being bullied online as well could bring additional suffering and harm. Online, the perpetrator of the abuse can be anonymous – much harder to pull off in real life – and this might add to the degree of distress it generates. Online, a single act of abuse can be endlessly replicated, spreading far beyond the victim's control. For young people in particular, the fact that bullying can continue online means there is no safe haven when the school day ends. Victims who feel unsafe at school now feel unsafe everywhere, whenever they pull out their phone. In this way, social media has enabled a new form of an old phenomenon that we already knew was damaging, and has potentially made it worse. But working out whether this really creates additional harm (traditional bullying is very harmful in itself) is a question for future research.

The public conversation

To summarise, then: social media is many different things at once, performing multiple functions even for the same person. For some, it can certainly be harmful. It can trigger and exacerbate existing vulnerabilities, and it can amplify and prolong social problems that started in the real world. Although we don't have definitive data on this, and possibly never will, it's entirely plausible that social media could be the trigger that tips a vulnerable person over the blurry line between mental health and illness. But social media can also be a source of a great deal of social support and joy, and it's vital that we recognise just how layered its effects can be. Those effects depend on a multitude of factors: a person's personality, their level of self-worth, their social or professional status, the apps they use, how they use them, the people they follow, the feedback they receive on their posts, whether they post at all ... even on what day it is. It's simply not possible to say whether social media is good or bad for mental health. It's both.

Yet the public conversation remains fixated only on the harms. I think part of the reason that social media has been so demonised boils down to one truth: it's new. There is an excellent website called Pessimists Archive, which posts old newspaper articles expressing alarm about technology and inventions we now use every day without much thought.[24] One 1897 article from the *Oshkosh Northwestern* describes an epidemic of 'telephone mania', saying that 'an unmistakable symptom of the disease is a desire to talk to people at distant points about all sorts of things at all hours of the day and night'. A 1944 *Pittsburgh Post-Gazette* article expresses concern about how radio is affecting young people's sleep: 'As every mother knows, often to her dismay – the radio causes a tremendous amount of friction between parents and children, and certainly presents a kind of obstacle to a smooth ending of the day, which parents were not faced with before this invention came along.' There are similar articles about the Sony Walkman, television and films. For all of history, people have been concerned about the latest trends in younger generations and the damage new technologies might be doing to them, fears that tend to abate as the generations pass and as different trends and technologies come along.

I also wonder whether there's something frustrating and scary for today's parents about being able to see so clearly how much psychological space their adolescent's social world takes up. Of course, some parents are worried about social media because their child is being bullied or has been upset by something specific that has happened online, and in that situation it's completely appropriate to be concerned. But in the absence of any stress or unhappiness, I wonder if there is just something unnerving about being able to explicitly see how much peers matter to young people – a social world that is now superseding that of the family, of the parents themselves. Peers and socialising have always dominated the lives of teenagers, but previously it was a little more hidden: contained in the mind, or expressed in parent-free spaces during and after school. Now, parents see this fascination manifest itself right in front of them. It's far easier to criticise and condemn phones than to recognise them for what they so often are: evidence of adolescents' entirely normal biologically driven social obsession.

Lastly, I wonder if some adults dislike social media for another reason: it is evidence of a stage of life they have left behind. There's a strange moment that all adults experience at some point when we realise that we are no longer the young ones. It was once us using the technology that grown-ups couldn't grasp, but now it's us who don't understand it. I'm reminded of a moment in *The Simpsons* when a young Grandpa says to his teenage son Homer: 'I used to be with it, but then they changed what "it" was.'

In truth, the fear and even contempt directed at social media probably stems from a bit of all of these things. To understand the recent increases in mental health problems and mental illness, it's reasonable to consider the effects of phones and social media. There really are some legitimate concerns about these platforms, and we still have very little decent evidence about their potential harms. But we shouldn't focus on phones and social media to the exclusion of other possible explanations. It is time to return to the question we posed at the start of this book. If we accept that increasing social media use is, at most, only part of the story, then what else might be contributing to the increased reported rates we're seeing today?

CHAPTER 8

Rethinking the crisis

In April 2020, Buzzfeed News published an article entitled 'Generation Freefall', written by journalist Ryan Brooks. He argued that the Covid-19 pandemic is just the latest of many hardships and insecurities faced by today's young people:

> Even if no one could have predicted the coronavirus pandemic, America's college students and early twentysomethings somehow aren't surprised. We were mostly toddlers and small children on September 11. Many of our first full memories of national news concern the 2008 financial crisis, the housing market collapse, and the subsequent recession that left many of our young parents in financial nightmares that stalled them for years.

The same argument has been made on this side of the pond. In an article for *UnHerd* published in April 2020, for example, politics professor Matthew Goodwin noted that by the time his current first-year university students turn twenty-five, they will have experienced two major financial crises as well as a global pandemic.[1] Goodwin, who was born in 1981, describes his own adolescence as one of relative hope and prosperity: a time of 'continuous economic growth, falling unemployment and expanding university education'. By contrast, the 'formative experiences' of Gen Z – those born between the mid-1990s and early 2010s – 'have included major economic downturns and recessions, international crises and divisive debates about the "losers of globalisation" and the rise of global populism'. He goes on:

> They were children when Lehman Brothers collapsed and the Great Recession followed. They were in primary school during the years of austerity, and in secondary school when the country voted for Brexit (a contest which they were not eligible to participate in). And today, after having already been set back by the Great Recession, they are preparing to graduate and enter the workplace just as a global pandemic sweeps across the globe and pushes the economy into yet another financial crisis.

This is partly why I find it utterly strange that so much of the discussion about young people's mental health is fixated on their phones: there's also been an awful lot of stress and disruption in the *outside* world for young people today and, as we know, all of this uncertainty and hardship are legitimate factors that could act as precisely the kind of external stressors that trigger mental illness. When trying to understand the recent increase in mental illness, self-harm and suicide, one plausible explanation could therefore be that there's simply more stress in people's lives now compared to those of previous generations.

Stress in the past

The trouble with this explanation is the implication that previous generations had it easier. It's beyond the scope of this book to give a historical rundown of every challenge and disruption that has been thrown at previous generations, but even limiting ourselves to the relatively privileged populations of the global north and west, the most cursory overview of the past hundred years, say, would include many wars, domestic and international terrorism, strikes and unemployment, financial crises and recessions, injustice and inequality. Arguably, it is the rule, not the exception, that each generation faces something that could be deemed a fresh and unique source of stress.

In 1881, for example, neurologist George Miller Beard published a book called *American Nervousness, its Causes and Consequences.*[2] In it, he described a new illness called *neurasthenia,* whose symptoms included 'fear of responsibility, of open places or closed places, fear of society, fear of being alone, fear of fears ... fear of everything'. He believed that a surge in cases of neurasthenia was being caused by dramatic social change caused by accelerating industrialisation, urbanisation and globalisation, the invention of offset printing, even trains – which meant everyone was now doing more and having to do it on a tight schedule. Modern life, in other words, was considered to be too stressful. An 1894 edition of *Harper's Monthly* stated: 'Something must be done – this is universally admitted – to lessen the strain in modern life.'[3] In the years that followed, journalists referred to 'our neurasthenia epidemic'.

The accounts of neurasthenia serve to remind us that the way we currently conceptualise mental distress is just one way of doing so, and that the names of disorders change across time. But they also remind us that almost every generation has its own set of stressors that they think are causing a unique breakdown in psychological well-being. They are related and similar to the cyclical fears about new technology. Yes, today's young people face a host of new challenges – especially in the context of Covid-19 – but it's not like previous generations grew up in environments that were easy. The nature of the stress was just different. So while there are indeed some new sources of stress, that can't be the whole story.

Coping, or not coping

In Chapter 5, we looked at how the way you interpret and cope with stress affects the likelihood that you'll develop a mental illness. Another possible explanation for the increase in mental health problems and disorders today is that we're exposed to the same level of stress – or maybe less stress – than people were previously, but we are *reacting* to it in a particularly bad way.

This argument is often inflated and oversimplified and used to blame young people for their distress. In 2018, for example, the *Sun* ran a story headlined: 'University bans litter pickers after snowflake students find them "stressful"'.[4] The following year, *Metro* ran a similar story: 'Students at the University of Oxford have voted to "replace clapping" with a silent wave because it "could trigger anxiety"'.[5] (The reason for the vote was more to do with students with autism spectrum disorder or hearing aids, apparently, but that nuance was missed once the story was shared online.) The tone of both these articles was one of mockery and derision, and this was only amplified in the resulting discussion on social media. At the end of December 2019, TV presenter Piers Morgan tweeted: 'As I keep telling anxiety-ridden snowflakes, we've never had it so good, so I hope 2020 is the year we start dwelling on the many positives of modern life rather than the negatives.' (Obviously, the tweet has not aged well.)

Like many people, I find these kinds of articles, and the term 'snowflake' itself, frustrating. It is often used by older people to criticise and shame the young, accompanied by wistful talk of Britain's stoicism of yesteryear: we used to be strong, is the implication, and now you are weak. The flaw in this logic is that you cannot blame a child for the way they've been taught to deal with stress. If a young person reacts 'badly' to stress, then that is surely the fault not of the young person but of all the adults and institutions around them who should help prepare them for life's challenges. But leaving blame and criticism aside, is there any truth in this argument? Are there *some* people who are coping less well, relative to their counterparts in previous generations?

One of the most thorough formulations of this argument was published in 2017 by US psychologist Jonathan Haidt and lawyer Greg Lukianoff in their book *The Coddling of the American Mind: How good intentions and bad ideas are setting up a generation for failure*. They put forward the thesis that American college students today are living in a culture of 'safetyism', in which feeling emotionally safe is of paramount importance. As a result, they campaign and protest to ensure that people they don't agree with are 'deplatformed' (prevented from speaking at events), or fired from their job, or shamed online. Collectively, this phenomenon is known as 'cancel culture'. Haidt and Lukianoff argue that increased mental health problems have led to this intolerance of disagreement and debate, and that in turn this intolerance makes students psychologically weaker.

Amongst other causes of safetyism, they point the finger at American parents. They argue that parents are now obsessed with safety, physical and psychological. As a result, many young people in college today have had childhoods devoid of any risk and therefore of any opportunity to learn how to be resilient. They present data that American children today, especially those in middle- and upper-class families, spend little time in unsupervised play, especially outside. Parents are now more likely to step in to help their children and to monitor their behaviour, right up to and through the college years. This parenting approach, Haidt and Lukianoff argue, gives children fewer opportunities to develop social skills and figure out their own solutions to problems.

Other academics have noted this phenomenon, and coined terms like 'helicopter parenting' (always hovering around children) and 'lawnmower parenting' (trying to solve children's problems for them and thus smooth the path in front of them). This is a relatively new approach to parenting, and it's logical that it may have made young people less equipped to cope when life inevitably throws up a challenge. Haidt and Lukianoff argue that 'overparenting', combined with schools and colleges that pander to these tendencies in students and parents, makes young people ill-equipped to deal with disagreements and stresses, and prone to protest against words and ideas they don't like. They draw a parallel with the rise in peanut allergies, in which well-intentioned policies that led to the banning of peanuts in schools ended up backfiring: a 2015 study showed that children with no exposure to peanuts were ultimately more likely to develop an allergy than those who had them as a snack several times a week.[6] Lukianoff and Haidt say the same thing is happening when we try and stop children being exposed to stress: 'Kids need to develop a normal immune response, not an allergic response, to the everyday irritations and provocations of life.'

I don't agree with everything put forward in the book. To my mind, plenty of the protests made by students in the US (and elsewhere) have been perfectly legitimate and necessary. But I do think they make a compelling case that *some* young people are overreacting to the level of threat in their environment, and that this may be fostered and encouraged – with the best intentions – by parents, schools and universities. If children are being taught that stress is something to be avoided at all costs, or handed over to someone else to deal with, then one can see how this could rob young people of important opportunities to learn to deal with stress themselves.

But the fact is that it's hard to know for sure. We know that, in general, people's ability to cope with stress improves during adolescence, meaning that adults tend to cope better than teenagers.[7] But we don't know whether young people today cope differently to their predecessors, because the necessary studies (which would need to track responses to comparable stressors in same-age people across different time periods) haven't been conducted.

Coping and self-harm

The evidence we do have relates to something more specific – and more troubling. As I said earlier in this book, people often self-harm because it's a means of managing overwhelming emotions. In 2019, Louis Appleby, the head of the National Suicide Prevention Strategy for England, said that more young people are now turning to this behaviour when they are in distress:

> If mental disorder appears to have risen over several years but self-harm & suicide have risen more steeply, that suggests

mental disorder has become more risky. That could happen if young people are increasingly seeing self-harm as a way of coping with stress and we have evidence that this is the case. This is dangerous because, as those young people, who have learned to view self-harm positively, get older, they reach age groups whose suicidal behaviour is more serious, more likely to be fatal. So there is a long-term risk that the current rise in self-harm in young people may lead to higher suicide rates in the future.[8]

The evidence he mentions – about more people seeing self-harm as a way of coping – comes from a study published in 2019 that analysed data from the Adult Psychiatric Morbidity Survey, a large cohort study of sixteen-to-seventy-four-year-olds living in England.[9] Over 6,000 participants were asked about self-harm behaviour in 2000, 2007 and 2017. It's the same study I described in Chapter 1 that shows rates of self-harm are on the up – and the participants who reported self-harming were also asked two specific questions about *why* they did it.

The first question was whether they self-harmed to 'draw attention to your situation or to change your situation'; the second question was about coping with emotions – whether they self-harmed 'because it relieved unpleasant feelings of anger, tension, anxiety, or depression'. Participants could answer yes to one, both or neither of the questions. The authors recognise in the paper that giving only these two options may have been a bit limiting – there wasn't scope for participants to give other explanations. Nonetheless, what they found is important.

Both motivations increased across time: at each time point, of all the people reporting self-harm, there was a higher percentage of people endorsing each of the motivations. But the coping explanation increased the most, particularly in females. The number of people self-harming in an attempt to draw attention to or change their situation roughly doubled between 2000 and 2014; the number doing it to relieve feelings of anger, tension, anxiety or depression approximately tripled. So this is one potential explanation for the rising rates of self-harm at least: that young people in distress now are more likely to use self-harm as a (dysfunctional) tool to cope with that distress. And as Appleby said, this is concerning not just in and of itself but because self-harm is a risk factor for later suicide.

The question then is this: w*hy* are young people expressing their distress in more physical ways now?

Social contagion of self-harm and suicide

Nobody has the answer to this yet, and there won't be one single explanation, but one relevant factor is that young people are discovering self-harm content online, and that this might trigger this behaviour. We have seen that adolescents care a lot about what their peers are doing, and it could be that social media is allowing them to learn more about this type of behaviour – leading them to try it out for themselves.

The fear of self-harm being 'contagious' isn't new: in 1968, psychiatrist P. C. Matthews published a paper in which he described an 'epidemic' of self-injury in an adolescent inpatient unit.[10] He observed that of the eleven patients who self-harmed over a seven-month period in the unit, ten of them said they had been directly influenced to do it by seeing or hearing about other patients self-harming. Many studies have since described the same phenomenon. An article published in 2013 reviewed sixteen studies that looked at potential social contagion of self-harm, from both community (school and college) and inpatient populations, and found that all sixteen studies showed that some people self-harmed at least in part because they had been influenced by this behaviour in others.[11] There are many things that lead a person to self-harm, but this is one factor that bumps up your risk: if you have a friend who self-harms, you are more likely to do it yourself, compared to if you had no self-harming friends.

This is relevant for suicide too. The notion of 'imitation' or 'copycat' suicide has been used to explain the occasional occurrence of suicide 'clusters', when for example several people take their own lives in the same school or town in a relatively short amount of time. Suicide clusters are more common in young people.[12] Copycat self-harm and suicide could be due to the fact that people who are already vulnerable are more likely to be friends with one another in the first place – this is known as *assortative relating*. Or it could be that having a friend who self-harms or (in particular) dies by suicide is intensely distressing, which acts as a trigger for or escalation of a person's own mental distress. But clusters can appear among people who aren't friends. It could be that learning about self-harm or suicide either in your friendship group or simply your local community provides information about means of doing it and/or normalises this behaviour.

Researchers Jill Hooley and Joseph Franklin examined the question of why most people *don't* self-harm.[13] Beyond the three immediate and obvious 'barriers' – most people don't want to be in pain, are squeamish about blood and wounds, and like themselves too much to hurt themselves – they proposed two further barriers that may serve to restrain those people for whom the first three no longer apply: most people just don't know much about self-harm, so it wouldn't enter their head as an option, and there's a strong social norm that self-harm is unacceptable. Once a person starts seeing and hearing about other people self-harming, especially friends, both these barriers break down.

So this is one possible explanation for the increased rates of self-harming among young people: greater access to the relevant information online. The more people who post and share this content, the more that information spreads and normalises the behaviour. But right now, we don't know for sure.

What else is going on?

We have considered three explanation thus far: young people are experiencing more stress than previous generations, coping less well with that stress, or learning from one another to cope with it in more physical and harmful ways. Clear evidence that would allow us to tease apart these possibilities is lacking, and it's possible that all of them are playing a role. But there are still many other possibilities worth considering.

One is that rates of mental illness may be getting worse because it might now be harder to get access to treatment than it has ever been in the recent past, meaning that people's distress escalates. In the UK, there have been cuts to the funding of mental health services. Data released at the start of 2020 showed that hospital admissions for eating disorders in the UK have risen considerably: from 14,000 in 2016–17 to 19,000 in 2018–19. If you have an eating disorder, you only get admitted to hospital when things are very severe – when your condition is life-threatening. There will be many factors contributing to an increase in hospital admissions but one of them could be that people are not getting the right help in the earlier stages of the illness. Ian Hamilton, a mental health academic in the UK, writes that funding cuts have played a role in increased rates of suicide: 'The cruel paradox is that as we have improved detection and acceptance of mental health problems like depression we have squeezed treatment budgets – we have fewer specialist resources than ever. This mismatch must have contributed to the surge in suicides.'[14]

Another point is that in the last couple of years, in England and Wales, the threshold for which a death is recorded as a suicide has changed. Before 2018, coroners needed to use a 'criminal standard' of proof: they had to consider that the death had been a suicide 'beyond all reasonable doubt'. In July 2018 the standard of proof was changed to the 'civil standard', meaning that coroners needed to consider on the 'balance of probabilities' whether a suicide had taken place. In cases where it's not clear whether a person intended to take their own life or whether the death was an accident, a suicide is now more likely to be recorded. In 2019, the Office for National Statistics wrote: 'It is likely that lowering the standard of proof will result in an increased number of deaths recorded as suicide, possibly creating a discontinuity in our time series. With the data in this release, it is not possible to establish whether the higher number of recorded suicide deaths are a result of this change.'[15]

There are yet more ideas. In 2004, the Food and Drug Administration in the US published a warning that in some children and adolescents, antidepressant use was actually linked to an increased tendency for suicidal thoughts and behaviour in a minority of patients. As a result, antidepressant prescriptions for these younger age groups fell considerably – which meant that some people who might have needed these drugs weren't getting them. This led to concern that the FDA warning might have inadvertently caused suicide deaths, likely more than it had prevented.[16]

Researchers have also drawn a link between the opioid painkiller epidemic in the US and the increase in youth suicide. One study from 2019 of nearly 150,000 children looked at medical records for opioid prescriptions in parents and for suicide attempts in children aged ten to fifteen. They found that children whose parents used opioids for more than a year were twice as likely to attempt suicide, compared to those whose parents who used none.[17] The absolute numbers were still low – 0.14% compared to 0.37% – but opioid addiction is increasing, so this could be one factor in the increasing rates of teenage suicide.

There is an awful lot going on here. Rates of mental illness, self-harm and suicide may be increasing for a combination of all of the reasons considered thus far. But there's something else I want to consider now – something that I think is happening in parallel with all of the above.

Has the changing mental health conversation played a role?

In Chapter 1 we established that pre-pandemic rates of mental illness were increasing, but perhaps not as rapidly as had been widely assumed. Recall also that much of the data that led to this conclusion derives from community-based studies conducted using questionnaires and interviews. As we saw, it's generally better to rely on these studies than on those that show an increase in the number of people actively seeking treatment, because the latter could simply be because people are now more willing and able to admit to their psychological difficulties. But in fact, this phenomenon could be playing a role even in the questionnaire and interview studies. This is surely a good thing, and the whole point of all those destigmatising campaigns: to ensure that people are now more confident about ticking the box that says they're struggling, or saying yes when the interviewer asks about possible symptoms. Therefore when rates of mental illness appear to have increased, that doesn't necessarily mean the *underlying* levels of distress are actually changing. It may be that – in part at least – people today are simply more willing to admit to problems that people in previous generations always had but wouldn't discuss, not even on an anonymous questionnaire.

This would be an entirely good thing. We need to remove the shame and secrecy that still surround so much mental illness. They make symptoms that are already frightening and debilitating even worse, prolong suffering, and in some cases, can be fatal. But of course, this increasing openness is going to change our perception of how common these problems are. The more people talk about mental illness – to their doctor, to researchers, to each other – the more it's going to seem like rates are increasing. We're just going to have to accept that as an unavoidable side effect of this important fight to reduce stigma.

Simultaneously, as we saw in Chapter 2, the official DSM guidelines that define mental illness have expanded rapidly over the last seventy years. Experts in the field have officially deemed that more and more phenomena should fall under the umbrella of mental illness, and this will have inevitably trickled down to the way we all understand our experiences. The lens through which we see our mental distress has been transformed – thanks to the official guidelines and the destigmatising campaigns – so that today we are more inclined to label milder or more transient psychological experiences as being within the realms of a problem or disorder. Not only are people now more willing to talk about previously hidden mental health problems and illness – what people understand 'mental health problems' and 'mental illness' to be has changed.

The upshot is that a person filling out a questionnaire about their mood in 2020, for example, will have a totally different cultural framework in which to understand what the questions mean. A person who scores 8/10 on a depression questionnaire now isn't necessarily more depressed than a person who scored 5/10 on the same questionnaire twenty years ago; they just have a different awareness of their psychological well-being, a different interpretation of the language being used.

Answers to questionnaires (and interviews, in fact) are entirely dependent on how respondents understand and interpret the questions, which in turn will be affected by the way in which those terms are discussed and defined and endorsed within their society. The Canadian psychiatrist Stanley Kutcher says it's essential to bear this in mind when we interpret any studies using self-report questionnaires of mental health symptoms over time: 'Youth self-reports of negative emotions are increasing, but the self-report scales used in studies documenting this have not been calibrated for generational changes in language use.'[18] In other words: we have no idea if, say, 'feeling down' means the same thing to a twelve-year-old today as it did to a twelve-year-old even a decade ago. But if we're now telling people that their negative feelings are noteworthy and something they need to address, then it makes sense that they might be more likely to think a questionnaire item like 'I've been feeling down' applies to them. The upshot could be many more people saying (and believing) they have certain problems, when nothing has actually changed.

Looping effects

The Canadian philosopher Ian Hacking is interested in why new labels for human experiences appear. In particular, he has argued the case for 'looping effects' – that labels can become somewhat self-fulfilling: 'I have long been interested in classifications of people, in how they affect the people classified, and how the effects on the people in turn change the classifications.'[19]

Psychologist Nicholas Haslam has applied the idea of looping effects to the concept of mental illness.[20] He argues that when professionals classify and name something as a mental disorder, they don't just describe something that already existed, they actually invent something new: that category, that thing, comes to life. People then come to recognise themselves in that label, and the concept becomes solidified. This in turn adjusts how they view themselves, according to what they learn about the label. As Hacking says, 'Our sciences create kinds of people that in a certain sense did not exist before.' Then – and this is the looping bit – the way in which people take on and embody these labels *influences the professionals*. They do more research on it, or they adjust and refine their thinking based on what they now see in the people who present with this disorder. Haslam sums it up: 'Changing ideas change people ... and changed people necessitate changes in ideas.'

Take binge eating as an example. Consider when academics and clinicians noticed that some people binge eat in a harmful and problematic way but they don't purge as someone with a typical case of bulimia would do. This was how the term binge-eating disorder came to be a separate disorder in DSM-5. But then people started being diagnosed with this disorder, or they started reading up about it and diagnosed themselves. Through that process, the reality of binge-eating disorder as a real entity in the world becomes confirmed. People go to their doctors saying they have binge-eating disorder, and researchers recruit people with those criteria for studies, and the iterative process between concept and person continues.

Haslam suggests that this same looping effect is also happening at a grander scale in society with the general concept of 'mental disorder', such that it has become an 'ever-expanding vortex'. As psychiatrist Derek Summerfield wrote in 2001: 'The constructs of "psychology" or "mental health" are social products. Collectively held beliefs about particular negative experiences are not just potent influences but carry an element of self-fulfilling prophecy; individuals will largely organise what they feel, say, do and expect to fit prevailing expectations and categories.'[21]

In other words, part of the reason why rates of mental illness seem to be rising could be because at a societal and cultural level, we are more readily interpreting our experiences as such. Through our language and interpretation, we may be *creating* additional cases of mental illness. The Hungarian-Canadian sociologist Frank Furedi refers to this as the 'problematization of emotional life', and that this has 'widened the definition of harm to a historically unprecedented point'.[22] Of course this can only ever be part of the explanation, and it is not a criticism of anyone who is experiencing mental illness or distress. As I say throughout this book, and as I know personally, these experiences are real and can be disabling, whatever we call them. But as a contributing factor to the phenomenon of rising rates, it is too plausible to be ignored.

Reported rates of mental distress and illness were rising before the pandemic, but was mental distress and illness *itself* increasing? The honest answer is that we don't really know. Many more people were certainly seeking help for these problems and receiving antidepressant medication. According to the best-quality research using questionnaires and interviews, the number of people experiencing mental distress and mental illness was increasing. Increased rates of self-harm in adolescent girls were especially pronounced, and rates of suicide were also increasing. This could all be for a host of legitimate reasons, many of which I have laid out in this chapter. But – suicide rates aside – it could also be that people are just talking about this more: thanks to the movement to destigmatise mental illness, more people are admitting to problems that were previously hidden, and getting them diagnosed. Finally, the shift in language around distress, particularly the ever-expanding boundaries of mental illness, could mean that more phenomena – some inappropriately – are now being labelled as mental disorders and problems. In truth, it's probably a bit of all of this.

What is certain is that, whatever the effects of the global pandemic, all of these factors will play a role in any subsequent increase in mental disorder that we see. And given that is the case, what might be done to better help people across the spectrum of mental health and illness? The final part of the book examines the treatment of mental illness – and mental health – and begins by looking more closely at the language we use, and whether in some cases that might be exacerbating some of the problems that we face. Because it was this very question that made me – as a person with a history of mental illness, as a lecturer supporting young people – want to write this book in the first place.

CHAPTER 9

Language matters

In 2018, Hannah Jane Parkinson wrote an essay about mental illness entitled 'It's Nothing Like A Broken Leg', which won her Mind's journalist of the year award.[1] In it, she wrote about her bipolar disorder, being sectioned, and spending time in psychiatric hospitals – and what she thinks about the current public awareness of mental health:

> In recent years the discussion around mental health has hit the mainstream. I call it the Conversation. The Conversation is dominated by positivity and the memeification of a battle won. It isn't a bad thing that we are all talking more about mental health; it would be silly to argue otherwise. But this does not mean it is not infuriating to come home from a secure hospital, suicidal, to a bunch of celebrity awareness-raising selfies and thousands of people saying that all you need to do is ask for help – when you've been asking for help and not getting it. There is a poster in my local pharmacy that exclaims, 'Mental health can be complex – getting help doesn't have to be!' Each time I see it, I want to scream.

In the next chapter, we'll see that it is often difficult to get access to treatment for mental illness, and when you do, it can be a long, unpredictable path to getting better. But Parkinson is expressing a more general frustration with the way we talk about mental health. She is saying that well-intentioned campaigns might actually be alienating the very people they are supposed to help, and I agree with her.

At the start of this book, I argued that we need to preserve the difference between mental illness and the psychological suffering that is a normal part of human experience, for the sake of those who are seriously unwell. But I've then spent a great deal of the book showing that there isn't a clear boundary between the everyday and the pathological. All symptoms – mood, worry, disordered eating, self-harm, delusions – everything exists on a spectrum. Along each spectrum, every psychological problem shifts gradually from being mild and controllable to something that can entirely take over your life. There is no sudden change, no distinct shift on any graph that indicates mental illness has begun. In addition, the processes that make a person susceptible to mental illness in the first place – genetic vulnerabilities, stressful life events, coping styles – are the very same ones that make a person susceptible to experiencing non-pathological distress as well. As we'll see later, the same applies to treatment: many treatments for mental illness are the very approaches that can help us all cope with other forms of psychological difficulty and distress.

And yet in this chapter I'm going to make the case that we do need to try, in the language we use, to maintain the distinction between health and illness nonetheless. Just because something's a spectrum, and there will be grey areas, doesn't mean we should use the same language for everything. We need to preserve some words – and a clear understanding of what they mean – for the people who are seriously psychologically unwell, even if the edges around that group are blurred. If we don't, everyone ends up suffering more.

This is emphatically not the same as ignoring or belittling other negative feelings. Even reasonably mild anxiety and mood problems can be exhausting. If you go through a period of stress like bereavement or prolonged illness, the psychological effects can be devastating. None of this is to say we should keep quiet about distress that doesn't meet the threshold of a disorder.

Quite the opposite. We need to talk about the psychological phenomena that cause us unhappiness or concern. Not just because they are unpleasant in themselves, but because they can be a warning sign, a red flag that someone is on the road to a more serious problem. This is what the current public conversation is getting right: we should talk about all this, take steps to look after ourselves when we're having a tough time, and reach out to people who we think might be struggling.

But one problematic consequence of the bid to destigmatise mental illness, and to recognise everyone's struggles, is that we've started labelling too much that is negative or distressing as a problem or disorder. This is particularly true of anxiety and depression. In August 2020, several months into the Covid-19 pandemic, Michelle Obama said on her podcast: 'These are not, they are not fulfilling times, spiritually. I know that I am dealing with some form of low-grade depression. Not just because of the quarantine, but because of the racial strife, and just seeing [the Trump] administration, watching the hypocrisy of it, day in and day out, is dispiriting.'[2]

I'm not disputing the seriousness of the context she describes, or questioning the idea that it could affect mood and sleep, as she goes on to say. I'm not questioning that these circumstances could indeed trigger a mental illness like depression, or that someone of her social standing could develop depression (when she made these comments, some of the responses online were along the lines of 'what has she got to be depressed about?', which is deeply unhelpful). But I quote her here because I think her choice of language is so revealing. It may seem a small, even pedantic point, but I believe it is indicative of something that permeates public discourse: 'some form of low-grade depression' implies that she's not really talking about clinical depression, and she knows it, but nonetheless wishes to invoke the gravity of the clinical condition. She could have said she's struggling, that the current political and social climate are affecting her mood, her sleep, her motivation. But instead, she chose to use the words 'dispiriting' and 'low-grade depression' as if they were equivalent.

In response to her comments, the UK mental health magazine *Happiful* published an article entitled 'What is low-grade depression?'[3] In it, they say that what Obama describes 'shares similarities' with a depressive disorder called dysthymia. This disorder involves relatively mild symptoms of depression that last for a very long period of time – according to the DSM-5, a person must experience low mood 'for most of the day, for more days than not', as well as at least two other symptoms like insomnia or poor appetite, for *at least two years* to meet a diagnosis. They do note this duration in the *Happiful* article, but the headline and overall tone imply that what Obama describes *is* a form of depressive illness, one for which a name must be found. They, too, reinforce the idea that experiencing some of the symptoms of a disorder is equivalent to experiencing the disorder itself.

This false equivalence is common now, such that for many people, perhaps the majority, it barely registers as strange. I recently asked a third-year undergraduate psychology student about how she and her peers discussed their mental health. She said *everyone* in her year group – more than a hundred students – self-identified as having depression or an anxiety disorder or both. From everything we know about population-based studies, it's nigh-on impossible that every one of them had a diagnosable mental disorder. The far more likely explanation is that some of them are liberally applying the psychiatric terminology that is now commonplace in our culture to more transient or low-level unhappiness or worry.

In 2004, US researchers conducted in-depth interviews with twenty-two teenagers (aged fourteen to nineteen) who had a diagnosis of depression.[4] The purpose of the study was to get a more detailed understanding of what teenagers thought about their experience of the disorder: what they thought started it, how they sought help, how they managed their symptoms. One particularly revealing section of the paper describes the point at which participants considered themselves to be depressed – the point at which they realised they were no longer experiencing 'normal' teenage moods, which the researchers refer to as 'funks' (emphasis added):

> If [the participants] were attempting to normalize their experiences by comparing them to those of other teens, this strategy eventually ceased to be effective, either because symptoms could no longer be characterized as 'normal' (e.g., suicidal thoughts) or because the duration of the funks became too long to be easily dismissed. *Teens eventually began to consider depression as a possible explanation for their experience* and then took action to help them decide if they were actually depressed by talking to friends or family members.

Of course, many teenagers still have the experience described here: they are depressed and don't recognise what is happening, or don't want to admit it. They don't seek help for mental health problems because of the stigma involved or because of a lack of awareness of their own symptoms.[5] Only eventually do they 'consider depression as a possible explanation'. But in the years since that 2004 study was conducted, the readiness with which we label low mood as depression has been transformed. There are now other young people – like some of those undergraduate students above – who reach for the word 'depression' as a first port of call, framing all experiences of low mood with this language.

Those who are most unwell

I appreciate this may sound very picky. Language is continually evolving through use, and ultimately any attempt to prescribe or control the meaning of words is at the mercy of that process. But as any lawyer, politician or diplomat will attest, language matters enormously. Calling everything anxiety and depression serves no one.

Most obviously, the expansion of mental illness terminology undermines the experience of the people who are most seriously ill. These are the individuals whose symptoms have become so intense and overwhelming that they cannot function in their life, causing immense distress and significantly impacting their relationships and their ability to work or to go to university or school; the people whose symptoms may be putting their lives at risk. 'To conflate normality and pathology devalues the currency of true illness.' There was barely even a public discussion about mental health when psychiatrist Derek Summerfield wrote these words in 2001.[6] His point is more important now than ever.

Within that cohort of students I described above, there definitely will have been some who have clinical depression. But in a context where everyone is depressed, how do they get their voice heard? If a student approaches their personal tutor or friend saying they have depression, that person may easily be thinking to themselves: *Yeah, who doesn't?* As a lecturer, I found that the sheer volume of students who self-identified with these problems made it very hard to distinguish what level of help was needed for whom. If every low mood is described as depression, if every psychological difficulty is framed as a mental illness, then we risk losing sight of the people who are truly ill.

If we describe everything using psychiatric terminology, another risk is that people will become sceptical of mental illness itself. The unhelpful language of 'snowflakes' is an example of this. If we refer to anxiety when we talk about students who are upset about campus litter, say, then some people may well conclude that this is what mental health problems really are: fragile young people complaining too much. Tabloid papers know this language is inflammatory; that's why they use it – and why the rest of us should not.

No language left at the top

Understandably, a form of linguistic inflation is now taking place, as a result of the overuse of psychiatric terminology.

Simply saying you have depression or anxiety is no longer enough to get noticed in the sea of mental distress. Many people will now say that they have *severe* mental illness in order to be taken seriously. In 2020, for example, the actor Alex Winter discussed the 'extreme PTSD' he experienced after being sexually abused as a child.[7] But PTSD *in itself* is extreme. There is no mild version. Or take this related example from a blogpost, in which someone describes their experience of loss:

> I cycled through every one of the Kubler Ross [sic] model's stages of grief several times. And as anyone who has been through the five stages of grief knows, they are not really stages at all, but rather suggestions. Grief is a full body contact sport that involves cycling and recycling through the stages of grief, moving forward and backwards and sideways at the most inopportune moments until the heart and soul decide there's nothing more to be done and they've let go. There's nothing rational about grief and no timetable to 'get over it'. It's insanely confusing and consumes massive amounts of emotional resources. Grief is involuntary and wild and frightening.[8]

Fair enough, you might think. But this is not a description of the writer's reaction to a death. It was about leaving a career in academia. The first sentence of this paragraph is 'The grief I felt when I conceded defeat on the job market was the real deal.' It is unfair to single out any individual and I certainly don't underestimate how hard it is to lose one's career or how keenly this writer felt it. But we have a responsibility to preserve the language of bereavement from devaluation. What about the people who really are in the quagmire of grief, trying to deal with the loss of someone they love?

We're giving the wrong advice to vulnerable people

A further consequence of this linguistic inflation is that we can end up giving the wrong advice to people who are in need of medical help and long-term support. Consider this extract from an essay on mental health by the comedian Miranda Hart, entitled 'Hello, My Loves':

> The condition with which you might have currently been labelled is not who you are. It will lift, but for now it is your superpower. It's your agency to change. It was mine. It was for anyone else I know who has gone to the depths of the cave where the treasures are to be found. You are a warrior for going in. The avoidance of feelings is the coward's way out, not the other way round and reframing your suffering as your superpower might just help you realize how strong you are, and what you can and will do with the unique treasure that you find on the brave journey through the darkness.[9]

It's hard to convey how much this passage clashes with my own experience of mental illness. The anxiety disorder and depression I experienced were not superpowers. There was no treasure to be found. The cave I fell into was dark and empty and cold, and it took a long, long time to find my way out. The primary thing my experience taught me was that mental illness is a horrible waste of time, energy and life. I'm not proud of the experience. I'm not ashamed of it either: it just *is*, it just happened.

Again, it is unfair to single out Hart here. The whole tone of the essay is warm and supportive and clearly comes from a good place, and she's certainly not the only person who has put this positive spin on mental illness; she's not the only one to call it a superpower. Rather, this is part of the 'positivity and memeification' of mental health that Parkinson describes. As the conversation around mental illness has mushroomed, so too have the cheerful books and pithy social media posts containing motivational mottos like 'Don't look back, you're not going that way' and 'Be your own reason to smile'. But this kind of message is not actually helpful to those in the gritty depths of a disabling disorder. In fact, it can be infuriating. And worse, it can misrepresent the reality of mental illness to those who have not experienced it – leaving sufferers misunderstood, again, out in the cold while those with more palatable problems support each other around a warming fire. 'Mental illness is ugly and my behaviour because of it has sometimes been ugly,' the writer Bryony Gordon tweeted. 'Until we acknowledge this, there is a long way to go.'

Overmedicalising doesn't help the individual

All of the downsides discussed so far affect those who are seriously unwell. But I'm not convinced that the inflation of language actually helps people with other forms of psychological distress either. Framing milder symptoms or the intense but normal suffering in response to life events as a mental illness – or even just as a 'mental health problem' – might be validating for some, but it will be disempowering and frightening for others. These words can create a sense of paralysis and victim-hood that does nothing to help the person who is struggling.

Even in people who are clearly ill, receiving a diagnosis of a mental disorder is a double-edged sword. When researchers ask people with mental illness how they feel about their diagnostic label, the response is mixed.[10] Some people report positive outcomes: finally having a name for their symptoms helped them understand their experiences and provided a sense of relief that they weren't making up their symptoms or imagining things. It confirmed that their problems were 'real', something that other people have experienced and documented. Diagnoses can also provide access to treatment and offer hope for getting better. But on the other hand, some people report that receiving a label of mental illness leads to hopelessness, disempowerment, stigma and discrimination. Many people feel these good and bad consequences in parallel.

I'm trying to extrapolate this to all the people now, particularly young people, who are framing their unhappiness as depression, their stress as an anxiety disorder, or any other difficulties as psychiatric illness. These people will now be more likely to think that their distress means there is something dysfunctional about their mind or brain. If this labelling acts as a doorway through which they gain access to help, then perhaps this is all worthwhile, but we need to think carefully about the baggage that comes with these labels when they may not be appropriate, and whether there might be other language we could use.

In Chapter 3, we saw that with the publication of the DSM-5, it became easier to get diagnosed with depression in the immediate aftermath of a bereavement. As I said, diagnosing a grieving person with depression has some potential benefits, such as greater access to treatment or support that might help, and in some cases a diagnosis is clearly necessary. But there's a downside too. If you tell someone who is grieving that they have a mental illness, when really they are experiencing a common and normal response to loss, then you potentially restrict their own ability to cope. You're telling them that the time-honoured means of managing grief – of time passing, of social support – may be less relevant to them, which could lead them to engage less in the very things that might help. You are also giving them, on top of their grief, the potential stigma that comes with a mental illness, and the challenge of processing what that means for them. Paradoxically, all this could end up making it harder for someone to get better.

Before my fully-fledged breakdown aged twenty, I had a period of prolonged sadness when I was seventeen, following the end of a relationship. There's no way to convey teenage heartache without it sounding trite, but it was an intense relationship that ended painfully, and it affected me deeply. I lost my appetite, I had trouble sleeping, I felt desperately sad. I continued with my life – I went to school, I saw my friends – but I thought about it constantly. I know now that I met some, maybe all, criteria for depression at that time. I know that if I was a teenager today, this label would almost certainly have been used, by me or someone else. Until recently, I lamented that that wasn't fully recognised at the time, because maybe I would have benefited from some additional support. But now I'm not so sure. I would certainly have benefited from some advice about navigating loss and looking after myself, but I think that labelling my feelings as depression would have done me more harm than good. Like every other teenager, I was ruminating on my identity then, trying to figure out who I was, and absorbing 'mental illness' into my fundamental fabric before I even hit eighteen could have been really unhelpful. I got over that heartbreak the way so many others do: by crying, by talking about it a lot, by gradually having fun with my friends. With the treacle-slow passage of time, it passed. Now I look back, I'm glad no one suggested I had depression, because on reflection I don't think I did.

None of this is straightforward. As we have discussed throughout this book, life events like relationship breakdowns really do trigger depressive episodes in some people, and in a lot of cases labels and professional help is absolutely warranted. But it's messy, because in parallel there are plenty of people who are desperately unhappy after break-ups and that's 'all' it is: a period of deeply difficult – but very human – sadness. And I don't think there's much room in society to just be sad right now.

Today's paradox

While writing this book, I attended a public debate at King's College London: 'Is PTSD being overdiagnosed?'[11] Psychiatrist Andrew Johns and epidemiologist Sharon Stevelink spoke in favour of the motion; academic psychiatrist Stephanie Lewis and forensic psychologist Gerard Drennan spoke against it. Both sides made compelling arguments, backed up by plenty of evidence. Those in favour described some of the points I've made so far in this book: that the term 'trauma' has been expanded, probably too far, and that a label of PTSD now seems almost inevitable after a negative event. Those against the motion described the many people who clearly had PTSD but weren't being diagnosed: people who desperately needed help but weren't getting it. I left with a clear conclusion: both sides were right.

Therein lies the strange paradox we face right now, with all disorders. We are overdiagnosing mental illness, coating too many types of distress in psychiatric language, but the confusing thing is that *we are also underdiagnosing* some cases. So much devastating mental illness is still going unmanaged and untreated. In the UK in 2018, 6,507 people took their own lives.[12] Even one single suicide is damning evidence that extreme distress is being overlooked. The fact that this number of suicides is in the thousands is a shameful indictment of our society's understanding of mental health, of the priority we give support services, of our collective ability to talk and to care.

In society right now, the most seriously ill people still don't have a voice. This is partly because these individuals are just too unwell: in the throes of serious illness, most people are not able to be interviewed, for example, or to advocate for themselves on Twitter. But it's also that severe mental disorders are still considered unpalatable and scary: we don't understand, and don't know how to respond to, a person who is hallucinating or starving themselves or planning to take their own life. The most distressing, debilitating disorders are being kept behind closed doors. As part of moving the conversation forwards, we need to make space for these voices to be heard. When people with severe mental illnesses cannot share their own experience, others need to help them do it, or advocate for them. This obviously includes more rare disorders like schizophrenia, bipolar disorder and OCD but it also needs to cover the disorders we think we understand: we need to communicate just how limiting and devastating depression and anxiety disorders are as well. Only then can we try and promote the distinction between these experiences and other forms of psychological distress and difficulty.

One way we can all help improve this situation is by being aware of the language we use. This will help to ensure that anyone having a hard time gets the right support, while the language of mental illness is reserved for those who truly need it. The first step is to allow space for normal human emotion in response to difficult events without labelling it as a disorder, even when that emotion is devastation. We should be comfortable talking about and responding to distress in its many forms – worry, loneliness, grief – without immediately resorting to a dictionary of disorders.

Second, we can all be more sceptical about what we read online and in the media about mental health. This is emphatically not to say we should treat a personal admission of mental illness with distrust, but rather to dig further behind any headline that deploys alarming statistics or makes sweeping generalisations. When specific research is reported, we should scrutinise what the researchers actually did and the definitions they used. Consider this headline to an article in the *Independent*, published in 2019, summarising research conducted by the charity Mind: 'Three in five secondary school pupils experience mental health problems'.[13] Three in five – the majority – sounds really bad. But what exactly do they mean by 'mental health problems'? If this term covers any negative feelings, like sadness and worry and irritability, then surely *five* out of five secondary students are going to experience mental health problems sometimes. To add to the confusion, the opening line states, 'Three out of five secondary school pupils have either experienced mental health problems themselves *or are close to someone who has*', which is an entirely different statement from the headline. And when you dig into the detail of the survey, it seems that the students were asked 'How is your mental health?' (which was not defined), and only 14% of the students answered 'poor' or 'very poor'. So it's not clear what, if anything, justifies the alarming three-in-five claim at all.

In July 2020, a few months into lockdown in the UK, several prominent Twitter users (including sports promoter Eddie Hearn) started tweeting the same message: it said 'Suicide figures are up 200% since lockdown' and included the phone number of the suicide prevention charity Samaritans UK. Within hours, thousands of well-meaning individuals had shared the message. But then people started asking the same question: what's the reference for this? It turns out there was no evidence it was actually true. Samaritans UK then posted their own tweet: 'There is currently no evidence of a rise in suicide rates. However we know that many people are struggling with their mental health during this difficult time and we're here 24/7 for whoever needs us. Thank you for raising awareness of our service to those who might need it.'

Maybe in this situation there was no great harm done – as the charity themselves said, it helped raise awareness of their services. But as we've seen earlier in this book, information about suicide can be distressing and dangerous for vulnerable individuals. Each of us can help by being cautious and sceptical when we share information about mental health, online and offline, and by always looking for sources.

The stories told from the top

The media themselves also have a role to play here. As is clear from examples in this chapter, newspaper articles can skew our understanding of our society's mental health. The journalist Mark Rice-Oxley says that the wealth of information we now have about mental health may be a contributing factor:

I think the data is part of the problem here. I have worked in a newsroom for thirty years and I know what gets editors up off their seats. They like to handle certainty, handle facts. This data revolution we've seen over the past twenty years has vastly increased the number of facts, statistics, datasets and metrics. But not everything that can be measured counts, and not everything that counts can be measured. This has also been overtly true of our efforts to quantify mental illness in our society. We should be very cautious about reading too much into those statistics because, if you go back to the research paper, the statistic is couched in quite a lot of caveats ... In general, in the media, you see how scientific papers can be flattened and simplified beyond recognition.[14]

You can understand why editors are in a bind: headlines must be short and clear, and shocking stories will always get more attention than ones that indicate a more complicated truth. But one simple way to improve things, which some publications already do, is to include a link to the original scientific study on which an article is based. This won't solve the problem entirely: for many scientific journals, only a brief abstract is available to view; the rest of the detail hidden behind a paywall. And of course, not everyone will have the expertise or motivation to read the specifics. But including such a link is at least a nod in the right direction, one that honours the original research and makes it slightly harder for true findings to be dressed up or disguised.

Or, as Rice-Oxley suggests, perhaps the media should rely a little less on the data altogether and more on reporting what mental illness is actually like:

> There is another completely different way of doing this story and most newspapers are already doing it. And that's to take the data out of it and tell the individual story. When you do that, you get some very successful pieces which explain what mental illness feels like and what it is ... I'd much rather see mental health covered that way, with numbers written into the middle of it with caveats – like 'A survey asked individuals if they felt they had depressive symptoms' rather than 'A quarter of the nation has depression'.

This is a two-way process: we need to be presented with better-quality information, and we need to be more careful consumers of it. And as we adjust and deepen our understanding of mental health, we need to gain collective confidence to include in these conversations full-blown mental illness, in all its exhausting reality. We need to share stories about what mental disorders really look like – our own stories, and, with permission, the stories of those we love. There are many brave people who have paved the way for this already, talking openly about the ongoing painful challenge of living with a mental illness, and we must keep it up. Only by keeping the stories coming can we hope one day to have a conversation about schizophrenia or bulimia, say, and for everyone in the room to understand what it is we really mean.

But of course, people with mental disorders need more than our adjusted words or our improved understanding. Many will also need professional help, and it's this part of treatment that I turn to next.

CHAPTER 10

Expert help

Many of the stories being published about mental illness involve people talking about how they suffered immensely and then recovered. These stories are extremely useful because they give hope and they offer advice and ideas to try, all of which are so important when you are unwell. But these stories can also give an unrealistic impression. Some people's experience of mental illness involves a one-off breakdown from which they eventually recover, but many people carry their illness with them long-term, sometimes for life. For some, their disorder will profoundly limit everything they might ever want to do or achieve. It might ultimately be fatal. For others, mental illness will be an unwelcome companion constantly occupying a corner of their mind: manageable, with enough effort and the right techniques, but ever-present. Or ongoing mental illness might be more like a ghost in the wings, faded until it's almost invisible, but always waiting to re-emerge in times of difficulty or stress. We need to expand our focus to include all these possibilities. We need to better understand what 'recovery' really means.

When you ask patients themselves what they expect from mental health treatment, they often don't expect their symptoms to totally disappear. No doubt everyone *wants* a simple cure, but most recognise that the treatments we have at the moment are not miracles. One study conducted in the Netherlands and published in 2020 held focus groups and interviews with people who had had treatment for depression, and the clinicians who gave the treatment.[1] Both groups were asked questions about what they felt were the most relevant and important outcomes from their treatment. Four key themes emerged from the patients' answers: they wanted to be able to perform and fulfil their normal social roles (like being a parent or going to work); to accept the illness and manage current symptoms; to have techniques to cope with depression in the future, should their symptoms resolve and reoccur; and to achieve personal goals, like improving self-esteem. The clinicians' responses were similar, except they also emphasised the importance of a drop in specific symptoms such as low mood and loss of pleasure, as measured by questionnaires. Everyone agreed that goal-setting was important: that parties should agree together the most important outcome of the treatment.

These findings indicate what so much treatment is about: it's about coping with and managing symptoms, not about making them vanish altogether. It would be really helpful if this were more widely recognised and acknowledged, because it would help to manage expectations and relieve pressure on individuals. For some people, mental illness is not something they 'recover' from, it is a long-term challenge and disability. It's a message that the friends and family of those who are ill need to hear too: sometimes, you're going to be in this for the long haul.

What does treatment look like?

Sooner or later, someone in your life – be it someone you love, a colleague at work, or a friend's partner – will need treatment for a mental disorder, and we all have a responsibility to understand roughly what that involves. People who don't have a disorder can also benefit from some of the approaches described in this chapter – for example, therapy can be helpful for someone who has suffered a bereavement – but its focus is primarily on those who need help for a disorder (or disorders).

In a best-case scenario, a person who suspects they may be ill would seek medical help and get an appointment with the right professional quickly. Let's say they go to a doctor and describe symptoms of a possible mental disorder – like they're crying all the time, or they're making themselves vomit after every meal, or they're too anxious to go out in public. What their doctor says next will depend on how severe the symptoms are, the resources available in the country or region where they live, and the doctor's own judgement and experience. The least intensive option will be some self-help advice – advice about exercise and sleep, for example, which we will consider further in the final chapter – and 'watchful waiting'.

If the doctor judges that they need more intervention than that, she may suggest medication or refer them for a course of talking therapy, like cognitive behavioural therapy (CBT). In the UK, waiting lists for intensive therapy can be dauntingly long, so alternatives such as very short-term therapy (just a few sessions), or CBT via apps or a computer, which is partially automated, might be offered first. For relatively straightforward problems, like panic attacks or phobias or mild depression, these light-touch therapies – without the need for medication – can be very effective. They teach the participant the general principles of psychotherapy, without the cost of a long-term course. If the person is more seriously unwell, they might be immediately prescribed medication or referred for more intensive therapy. If their problem is sufficiently severe, or they have a particular combination of symptoms, then their doctor might refer them to a more specialist service or psychiatrist. This could happen if they show symptoms of psychosis like hallucinations and delusions, for example, or if they have anorexia. These experts will then offer their own combination of medication, therapy and self-management.

The controversy of antidepressants

There are many classes of psychiatric drugs, which each have their own profile of benefits and risks, but the most common ones are antidepressants called selective serotonin reuptake inhibitors (SSRIs), such as sertraline and fluoxetine (brand name Prozac). 'Antidepressant' is a bit of a misnomer, in fact, because these drugs are used to treat other mental disorders besides depression, including OCD, bulimia and anxiety disorders. As noted in Chapter 1, the number of people taking SSRIs is increasing – in the UK, prescriptions have almost doubled in ten years, from 36 million in 2008 to 71 million in 2018. There is less stigma associated with their use: many celebrities, including Jim Carrey, Chrissy Teigan and Kirstin Bell have talked openly about taking them. It's now not uncommon for people to talk about psychiatric medication on social media. In 2020, an online campaign led by the UK charity Autistic Inclusive Meets encouraged people to share photos of their medication with the hashtag 'Show Us Your Meds'. But stigma around them hasn't disappeared.

For some, particularly if their pain is sufficiently acute and distressing, the decision to take antidepressants is straightforward. For others, whose symptoms burn slowly, and who are broadly still able to function in their lives, there may be more room for deliberation. Do they actually work? What are the side effects? Is it hard to come off them?

Antidepressants have taken a bit of a bashing in recent years. Studies have shown that newspaper articles are more likely to portray antidepressants negatively than positively; the reverse is true of psychotherapy.[2] This negative press is partly a result of a series of meta-analyses published by Irving Kirsch, a psychologist at Harvard Medical School. Kirsch was originally interested in the placebo effect – when someone's symptoms improve in response to what they believe to be a course of treatment but in which the active component is, in fact, absent. This powerful phenomenon has been widely observed across medicine, and Kirsch was interested in the role it might play in recovery from depression, since a key symptom of depression is hopelessness, about one's future and the depression itself. If seeing a doctor and starting medication gives a person hope, could that be sufficient on its own to pull them out of depression, regardless of what is actually inside the tablets they are taking?

In 1998, Kirsch and his PhD student Guy Sapirstein looked at nineteen studies that compared two randomly assigned groups of depressed people: one group who took antidepressants (which were sometimes SSRIs but sometimes other types of antidepressants) and one group who took a placebo.[3] In both groups, the pills looked identical, so the participants didn't know if they were in the drug or placebo group. Across studies, the researchers expected that depressive symptoms would drop in both groups – they expected antidepressants would work, but also that placebos would too, to some extent. This is exactly what they found. What they didn't expect was how small the differences in the two groups were. The people who received a placebo either recovered to the same extent as the active antidepressant group, or they fared only a little bit worse. This finding was supported by more studies in the late 1990s and 2000s, some of which Kirsch was involved with, and some of which he wasn't.[4] Since there was never much difference between the two conditions, the conclusion was that antidepressants largely work because they act as a placebo.

If antidepressants are just a placebo, then it's unethical to prescribe them, because of the potential risks involved in taking these drugs. Some people experience side effects, like sexual dysfunction, headaches and a dry mouth while taking SSRIs; others experience withdrawal effects when they come off them – such as restlessness, irritability and trouble sleeping. Because of this, there was and still is intense academic and media interest in the possibility that antidepressants are placebos. On the day that one of his studies was published in 2008, Kirsch said, 'I awoke to find that our paper was the front-page story in all of the leading national newspapers in the United Kingdom.'[5] In 2009 he published a book entitled *The Emperor's New Drugs: Exploding the Antidepressant Myth*.[6]

But in April 2018, a study led by psychiatrist Andrea Cipriani at the University of Oxford questioned the idea that antidepressants are just placebos.[7] It was a meta-analysis of an impressive 522 trials, with a combined total of more than 116,000 participants. The trials covered twenty-one different antidepressants, including some SSRIs but also other types of antidepressants. These researchers found that all twenty-one antidepressants studied were more effective than the placebo. The placebo response was still relevant – people on dummy pills saw an improvement too – but the active antidepressant drug gave a considerable added benefit, more so than earlier studies had implied. And because of the sheer size and quality of this new meta-analysis, academics and clinicians were much more confident in its findings. Others have criticised *these* findings by saying that the added benefit is still not large enough for the drugs to be worth the potential risks. But this is tricky: a small average effect across a large group of people doesn't mean the effect for everyone is small; while antidepressants may be ineffective for some, they can be incredibly helpful for others.

Right now, we don't know in advance who will respond best to these drugs, or which drug might work best for them. Camilla Nord, a neuroscientist who researches depression treatments, says, 'There are lots of different types of antidepressants, so it's not like someone is an "antidepressant responder" per se, but maybe there is one type of drug they will respond to, and others that they won't. But we don't really know why this is at all yet.'[8] Right now, unfortunately, medication for mental illness is largely carried out on a trial-and-error basis until the doctor and patient find something that works.

Therapy

The other main treatment option is 'talking' therapy, in which the patient meets with a psychotherapist to discuss their symptoms and the wider context of their life. It may be offered alongside medication, or as an alternative to it. The evidence suggests that having both treatments in parallel is most effective: a meta-analysis published in 2014 in the Netherlands, for example, showed that having antidepressants and CBT together was more effective than just having the medication, for major depressive disorder, panic disorder and OCD.[9] A 2020 meta-analysis of nearly 12,000 adults with depression found that combined medication and psychotherapy improved symptoms more than either treatment alone.[10]

Talking therapy provided by a public health service like the NHS will likely be time-limited (with the number of sessions set in advance) and manualised – that is, the therapist will follow a prescribed set of steps laid out in a manual. The type of therapy will often be CBT, as this is an evidence-based and cost-effective talking therapy. Underlying this approach is the idea that your thoughts (cognition) and behaviour affect how you feel, and vice versa. This fits well with the network theory of mental illness discussed previously – the idea that various symptoms can trigger and affect each other. To change how a person feels, they need to change the way they think and behave. For CBT to work, the patient needs to carefully decipher what their thoughts actually are, which means formalising them into specific statements such as, 'I'll never be able to hold down a job' or 'If I eat that biscuit I'm worthless and disgusting' or 'If I go to the party no one will talk to me'. This might sound straightforward, but it can feel pretty alien to start with, and for some people is nigh-on impossible. It's relatively easy to recognise that you feel down or hopeless or anxious, but harder to identify the exact thoughts accompanying those feelings.

The next step is to interrogate and scrutinise those thoughts, either alone or with the help of the therapist. Having figured out what the thought is, the person then needs to replace it with a more helpful one. To do this, they might need to think about what evidence there is for and against that thought, and whether there's an alternative, more balanced way of looking at things. One of the CBT exercises for managing worry, for example, involves asking oneself three questions: what's the worst that could happen, what's the best that could happen, and what's the most likely thing to happen?

Imagine a person with social anxiety disorder who is particularly anxious about public speaking, and who has to give a presentation at work. One of the specific thoughts he identifies is this: 'I'm going to mess up the presentation and embarrass myself in front of my colleagues.' In answer to the first question – what's the worst that could happen – he might say something like, 'My mind will go blank, I'll not be able to say anything at all, I'll have a panic attack, everyone will laugh at me and I'll never be asked to lead future projects.' To answer the second – the best possibility – he might say, 'The presentation will go really well, I'll remember everything without relying on my slides, I'll answer questions insightfully, and will impress my boss.' Finally, to consider the most likely possibility, he'd say something like, 'I might feel really anxious beforehand and stumble over a few lines, but I'll get through the presentation okay and no one will think differently of me.'

The idea with this exercise is that the individual gradually comes to realise that the thoughts they keep having are actually rather skewed, inaccurate representations of reality. For someone with an anxiety disorder, the worst-case scenario is the default. The worst scenario is the *only* scenario: it's what's going to happen. But the more they ask themselves the second and third questions – in theory – the more they realise that the imagined scenario is unrealistic. The most likely reality will be somewhere in the middle: a bit bad, perhaps, but never as bad as they imagine, and it could even be good. By adjusting their thoughts to include and eventually focus on a fairer and more balanced interpretation of the situation, in theory there will be a positive knock-on effect on how they feel and what they are able to do.

Cognitive exercises like this are accompanied by behavioural ones – the 'B' part of CBT. For someone with depression, this might involve scheduling simple activities to get them out the house or re-engaging with the world in some way, and then seeing how that affects their mood. (In fact, in a related type of therapy called behavioural activation therapy, a person would focus *exclusively* on exercises like this.) For someone with an anxiety disorder, the behavioural component involves setting up 'behavioural experiments' and 'exposure' practices with their therapist in which they safely try out challenging situations and monitor the effect they have on their thoughts and mood. A key problem with anxiety disorders in particular is that people start *avoiding* the things that might cause them anxiety, like going to parties or getting in lifts or driving on the motorway. This may help in the short run – less anxiety – but in the long term it means the anxiety is maintained, because they never learn how to cope in that situation or have the opportunity to discover that it's not as bad as they imagined it might be.

The idea is that the person tests out the things they're scared of in a limited and controlled way: what is known as *graded exposure*. If someone is extremely anxious about driving on the motorway, for example, their first behavioural experiment is not to drive up the M1 on their own. Instead, they would come up with a list of activities *related* to driving on the motorway, grade them in terms of how anxiety-provoking they are, and then start with the easiest. They might practise driving on a busy road with a friend, then build up to driving one junction of the motorway with them at a quiet time, then driving one junction on their own, for example. The very initial steps of graded exposure can involve looking at pictures or videos of the feared activity, or even writing down its name. The idea is that the person only moves on to the next activity once they feel comfortable with the current one, thus gradually and safely learning that what seemed so terrifying is actually manageable.

CBT is not for everyone. Some find it exceptionally helpful, but the truth is that changing the way you think is really, really hard. It can feel like the equivalent of trying to change your political or moral beliefs, or changing who you love. For this reason, it can be helpful to know that not all therapies take this analytic approach to thoughts. Mindfulness-based therapy, for example, does almost the opposite: the patient is told to not scrutinise or attach any great meaning to their thoughts but instead to let them just pass over them. A person undergoing this kind of therapy might be encouraged to envisage their thoughts travelling past them as though they are on a station platform and their thoughts are a passing train, or to view them as clouds in the sky. In behavioural activation therapy, as I mentioned above, there's not much focus on thoughts at all but instead on how your behaviour – particularly your daily activities – might affect your mood. Finally, 'depth' therapies, like the psychoanalysis invented by Freud, don't pay exclusive attention to the thoughts and behaviour of the present but instead focus a lot on events in the person's past that may have led to their present symptoms.

What approach works best?

There is no single type of talking therapy – therapists approach a person's difficulties in many different ways using many different techniques. Those who pay for their own treatment – which many people resort to when faced with long waiting lists – will be able to choose between different options. Many private therapists have a preferred specialism but offer a flexible approach, dipping into different techniques depending on what's most effective for each person and their particular problem.

There's some interesting evidence that it doesn't really matter *which* type of therapy you have; the outcome is likely to be the same. Meta-analyses have found that different types of psychotherapy result in the same level of symptom improvement, and this is true of various disorders including depression,[11] PTSD,[12] panic disorder[13] and OCD.[14] Could it be the fact of having therapy, rather than the specifics of therapy itself, is what helps? Proponents of the 'common factors' model of psychotherapy believe so and argue that there are a number of features that exist across all successful therapy, which are what drive positive outcomes.[15] One of the key common factors, for example, is the 'therapeutic alliance', the working relationship between therapist and patient and, specifically, the quality of their bond and the extent to which their goals for the therapy are aligned. Therapists who are flexible, honest, warm and open are more likely to have a decent therapeutic alliance with their patients, as are therapists who can accurately interpret and reflect the patient's thoughts and feelings back to them. But as in any relationship, it is not the individuals so much as the dynamic *between* them that matters; how much they 'click'. As the writer Bryony Gordon puts it: 'Finding a good therapist is like finding a good boyfriend or girlfriend.'[16]

Another common factor in successful therapy is that the person has a positive expectation that it will be useful for them. This will depend partly on the expectations they have before therapy starts, but also, again, on the therapist who will provide a rationale for why the person is experiencing their symptoms and what the path is to alleviate them. Whatever the therapist's proposed method may be, if the rationale they provide gives the patient *hope* that having therapy will help them get better, then it is more likely to do so.

Not all evidence supports the idea that common factors explain why good therapy works. First, not all studies have found every type of therapy to be equally helpful. And just because two therapeutic approaches are similarly effective, doesn't mean they're doing exactly the same thing, or that the approach they take doesn't matter. As psychologist Pim Cuijpers and colleagues point out in a review of the topic, 'Many roads lead to Rome'.[17] The debate about different approaches, and why exactly therapy works when it does, goes on. But all that notwithstanding, psychotherapy can clearly be a powerful tool in helping people manage and reduce the symptoms of mental illness.

Therapy, when you find the right person, is a strange and wonderful thing: the most intimate non-intimate relationship you will ever have. You open up your heart and mind to a stranger and they change, or save, your life. It's exceptionally rare to be fully listened to. Possibly for the first and only time in your life, you are given the opportunity for your most distressing thoughts or harmful behaviour or darkest fears to be truly heard, without judgement. There's a lovely cartoon drawing about therapy, where the patient or client has a speech bubble above their head containing a knotted tangle of multicoloured wool. The threads of wool travel across the room to the therapist in another chair, and in her own speech bubble, the threads have all been separated out clearly into balls of different colours. This is what a good therapist does: you throw out a mess of thoughts from the deepest corners of your mind and they warmly guide you through it all, in a way that somehow makes sense. But even that description doesn't quite explain it. What is special and rare about a therapist, relative to other relationships, is that they help *you* figure out what the problem is. They don't tell you what they think, or what you should think. Instead, they very gently help you work it all out for yourself.

The reality of trying to get help

This is what treatment looks like in an ideal scenario. But the sad reality is that the people who are able to access therapy are the lucky ones. Many people with mental disorders *try* to talk to a professional about getting help only to discover that help is not available. In the UK, there are so many people who would benefit from, or who desperately need, psychotherapy. But there's not enough NHS funding to cover it and they can't afford to pay for it themselves.

According to official NHS figures, in the year to July 2020, 87% of people waited less than six weeks for their first session of talking therapy, which on the face of it sounds pretty good.[18] But even six weeks is a *long* time to wait if you're experiencing a mental health crisis. A minority (5%) had to wait more than eighteen weeks to be seen – sometimes considerably longer, depending on where they happened to live.[19] On top of this, this figure disguises the issue of 'hidden waiting' that most people experience after the first appointment, which is invariably an assessment and diagnosis; treatment proper doesn't start until the second appointment. When you are in crisis, every day you're not getting help is horrendous; weeks or months can be life-threatening. This is why GPs are so often compelled to prescribe antidepressants: they have no other treatment to offer.

One study published in 2020 looked at over 21,000 referrals to specialist child and adolescent mental health services and found that 26% of young people were seen within two weeks; some were even seen on the same day.[20] But the average wait was seven weeks, and 7% of participants weren't seen for more than nineteen weeks; the longest wait was, shockingly, more than four years. It is a tragedy and a mess that talking therapy and specialist services are not sufficiently well funded and that people in need cannot get the right help quickly.

Effects of destigmatising campaigns

In 2017, the psychiatrist Simon Wessely said: 'Every time we have a mental health awareness week my spirits sink. We don't need people to be more aware. We can't deal with the ones who already are aware.'[21] He was criticised for these remarks but it is incontrovertible that we are funnelling more and more people into a system that's already overwhelmed, and with the looming impact of Covid-19, things may be about to get worse. In 2019, Channel 4 released a Dispatches documentary entitled *Young, British and Depressed*, which explored the reports of increased mental health problems in young people today. The documentary raised the possibility, as Wessely did, that the anti-stigma campaigns may be contributing to the problem. Jenny, a young person featured in the programme, said this: 'These campaigns are asking people to reach out for help, it's okay to feel this way, it's okay like there'll be help there if you reach out. There isn't. There isn't help. And so I actually think it's dangerous that we're telling people that and it's not the case.'[22]

The drive to get more people to go to their doctor will undoubtedly have been helpful in many cases. When people who are struggling can access treatment, it means less suffering and more saved lives. But when we tell everyone in distress to get help but do not match that with appropriate funding, we create two problems. One is that people who need medical help and are persuaded to seek it face the blow of finding it unavailable to them, potentially compounding their sense of isolation and hopelessness. The other is that, combined with the widespread misapprehension of what mental illness actually is, we drive people to seek medical help who may not actually need it, depleting scarce resources. The potential impact of this on the availability of treatment is truly scary, and utterly ironic, since the idea of these destigmatising campaigns was of course to get help to the people who needed it.

The obvious problem here is lack of resources. There is a serious underfunding problem, and more money is needed. But another remedy, alongside properly funding mental health services, is to promote the message that, for milder or more transient levels of distress, there are many things that people can do *themselves* to manage how they're feeling. This is what I turn to in the final chapter.

CHAPTER 11

Helping each other and ourselves

In 2019 I attended a conference about the mental health of university students in the UK. Most of the talks were by academics or university administration staff, but one talk was by James Murray, father of Ben, a student who had taken his own life at university the year before. James described how they had been for lunch together on the day Ben died, and Ben had given no indication to his dad that anything was wrong.

The talk was devastating and powerful. Compared to the distractedness and laptop tap-tapping that usually accompanies these talks, when James spoke, the room was utterly silent. And I really remember, in particular, one thing that he said. He implored university staff, especially personal tutors, to ask how their students were, and to not just do it once. He said don't just ask 'How are you?', ask 'How are you *really*?' It's a powerful message for time-pressed academics, who are often squeezing in student meetings amidst a pile-up of other teaching, research and admin demands. But it's such an important message for everyone.

At the end of the previous chapter, we touched on the unintended consequences of encouraging people to seek professional help that isn't always available. But mental health awareness campaigns also encourage us to speak to our friends and family when we're struggling – and this reveals a different kind of problem. It's hard to just come out and say you're suffering.

It's hard to be cooking dinner or watching TV and suddenly say: I feel so low and hopeless. I cut myself today. I think the neighbours are tracking our conversation. I'm making myself sick after I eat. I'm lonely. I'm scared. So one simple thing we can all do is make it easier for the people around us to talk about how they're feeling. Ask them how they *really* are. But we then need to know how to respond, and not enough of us do. Opening up isn't much help to anyone if it's met with a blank and awkward stare. In fact, seeking emotional support from someone who responds badly like this can easily make a person feel worse. Key to a more helpful response is knowing how to listen properly – what's known in the literature as *active listening*.

Active listening is important, and often explicitly taught, in many professions. In psychotherapy, of course, but also in education, medicine and social work. It is central to mental health and suicide-prevention phone lines like the Samaritans and Niteline. The exact definition of active listening varies depending on the context, but it broadly includes non-verbal and verbal behaviour that demonstrate attention, understanding and empathy for the speaker. Non-verbal aspects are simple: eye contact, nodding, a posture oriented towards the speaker. Verbal components include paraphrasing what the speaker has said and reflecting back their thoughts and feelings. An active listener might say things like 'So you feel like … ' and ask questions afterwards to check understanding: 'Does that sound right to you?' They also ask open questions to guide the conversation, such as 'How did that make you feel?' Anyone who has had (good) psychotherapy will know that therapists do this in spades, but everyone can learn and practise these techniques.

One study published in 2015 investigated the impact of active listening during informal helping conversations.[1] The researchers recruited 301 undergraduate students and asked them to discuss two stressful events they had recently experienced – such as academic challenges or relationship problems

– for five minutes with a randomly assigned partner. What the participants didn't know was that some of the partners had in fact been trained in active listening by the researchers. At the end of the five minutes, the undergraduates who had been paired with the active listeners were more likely to report that their partners had high levels of emotional awareness, and more likely to say that the conversation improved their mood. These techniques are surprisingly simple on paper but we often forget to listen like this, or aren't aware of how much difference it makes – when actually it's a key thing we could all be doing to help people who are struggling.

Another important and worthwhile thing we can do is to become familiar with how to talk to someone about suicide. When someone is depressed, people are often afraid to bring up the topic of suicide, for fear that doing so will 'put the idea' into the person's head or make them feel worse, but research has shown this isn't the case. In one study from 2005, for example, high-school students in New York State were asked to complete a questionnaire.[2] Half of the questionnaires included questions about whether the respondent had experienced any suicidal thoughts, and half of them didn't. Two days later, they all answered another questionnaire about depressive symptoms and suicidal thoughts, and there was no difference between the two groups in terms of the number of these symptoms reported. In fact, 'high risk' students (those who already had high levels of depressive symptoms or previous suicide attempts) in the suicide questionnaire group were actually better off two days later than their counterparts in the control group – they reported less distress and less suicidal ideation. A 2020 meta-analysis evaluated the impact of asking about suicide and self-harm in healthcare and community settings and found no harmful effects – they found asking these questions may even reduce psychological distress in some cases.[3] This is the message promoted by suicide charities: asking someone openly about possible suicidal thoughts is far more helpful than leaving them to cope with those thoughts alone.

The Australian charity Conversation Matters[4] and the UK charity Samaritans[5] recommend asking someone directly if you're concerned: have you been thinking about suicide? If the person says yes, they suggest the active listening techniques mentioned above. Open questions are recommended: 'How long has this been going on? Has anything happened recently that's made you feel worse?' They suggest listening to the person's response without judgement, reflecting back what they are saying ('It sounds like you've been feeling really low'), and telling them you value and care about them. If they say they have been thinking about suicide, the advice is to ask them about it in a bit more detail to ascertain whether they're in immediate danger – ask them if they've made any specific plans, like if they've thought about how and when they would do it, or if they've written a note, or taken any steps towards their plan.

Charities also recommend doing what you can to keep the person safe. They suggest staying with them if you are together in person, or staying on the phone. If you're concerned that they are at imminent risk of harm, contact emergency services – or call a helpline at any point for additional support. Alternatively, if they're not at immediate risk, the advice is to talk together, if you feel able, to work out who else they can involve and what else you can do. You could, for example, help the person book an appointment to see the doctor or call a helpline on their behalf. A professional can help them make a 'safety plan' – so they have ideas for what they should do if they feel suicidal again.

Supporting someone who has a mental illness or who is suicidal is really hard. If you are looking after someone, make sure you can turn to other people for support for yourself. And remember these words, shared widely online and ascribed to Stephen Fry, who was among the first and most prominent celebrities to speak openly about his experiences of mental illness: 'It's hard to be a friend to someone who's depressed, but it is one of the kindest, noblest, and best things you will ever do.'

Exercise

Supportive friends and loved ones are so important to someone coping with mental illness or going through a difficult time. But we can also all learn ways to help *ourselves* when we're struggling. Of course, medication and therapy from professionals are often needed too, and some people will need ongoing medical support; others will be too seriously unwell to be able to carry out these approaches, often referred to as 'self-help'. But for many others – and even those who do need medical care – there are simple, worthwhile and helpful techniques we can learn to look after ourselves.

Some of the best things we can do to manage mental illness don't actually involve tackling our thoughts and emotions directly, they involve the body. Think for a moment about the last time you felt low, even just a temporary bout of sadness: where did you feel it? Many people report feeling sadness not in the head, but in the chest.[6] When people are depressed, it's often experienced as a deeply uncomfortable *absence* of bodily feeling: a hollowed-out emptiness or detachment. We feel anxiety in our body too; panic in particular can take over the whole body. In his book *The Body Keeps the Score*, psychiatrist Bessel van der Kolk describes how fundamental the body is to the entire experience of trauma, and the key to recovery from it.[7] All this means that when we look for ways to support our mental health, we shouldn't just rely on therapist appointments or cognitive exercises to change our levels of distress. We should think about what we can do with our *whole body* to manage the way we feel. And one critical way of doing that is exercise.

There is now a wealth of evidence showing that exercise is helpful for preventing, treating and reducing relapse of mental illness. A meta-analysis published in 2014 found that physical activity reduced symptoms of depression and schizophrenia in adults.[8] A number of studies have demonstrated the beneficial effects of exercise on anxiety, both for relieving a temporary state of anxiety and for reducing symptoms in those with anxiety disorders. Benefits of exercise have been shown for adolescents,[9] working-age adults,[10] and older adults.[11]

There are many possible explanations for why exercise is so helpful. There is the oft-touted explanation that exercise releases endorphins, a type of neurotransmitter, which can relieve pain and induce feelings of pleasure and positive mood. There are other physiological pathways too – including reducing levels of the stress hormone cortisol – but there are also social and psychological factors to consider. For example, those who exercise with other people will have the added benefit of social contact and support, and there will be psychological effects such as an increased sense of self-worth, improvement in how a person views their body and appearance, and a sense of accomplishment as they learn a new skill or develop their abilities, all of which affect mood.[12] Considering the list of potential benefits, it's easy to see why exercise is now recommended as a treatment by the NHS for those with mild to moderate anxiety and depression.

Of course, this won't work for everyone. Some people will have physical health problems or disabilities that make exercise impossible, or their mental disorder might be sufficiently severe that they cannot find a way to start exercising, or that it won't be effective if they do. Fatigue – either as a result of medication or the disorder itself – can make exercise impossible. Finally, some disorders can lead to excessive exercise as a dysfunctional means of managing anxiety or, especially in the case of eating disorders, one's weight; in such cases, recommending exercise is obviously unhelpful.

But there are other ways the body can be harnessed to improve mental health. Popular among them is simply learning how to relax physically. Not the 'lie on the sofa with a glass of wine' kind of relaxing but actually training the muscles to release tension and reduce physiological stress. Relaxation training is particularly relevant for anxiety, and is often taught either as a stand-alone treatment or alongside medication and/or therapy. A review paper published in 2008 looked at four types of relaxation training in the treatment of anxiety.[13] The first was a simple technique called progressive muscle relaxation, in which you gradually tense and release different groups of muscles in your body. This technique was developed by medical doctor Edmund Jacobson in 1929 and is still used today.[14] The second was autogenic training, a series of six steps which aims to achieve muscle relaxation through repetition of a series of phrases, such as 'my right arm is heavy'. Applied relaxation, the third, is a broader programme that encompasses progressive muscle relaxation and encourages individuals to relax their body during daily activities. The fourth was meditation, which includes mindfulness. The authors found that, combining data from twenty-seven different studies, all types of relaxation therapy were helpful for anxiety disorders and anxiety more generally, particularly meditation. These approaches are not without their limitations – meditation can occasionally cause adverse effects such as panic attacks or re-experiencing of trauma.[15] But for many individuals, relaxing the body can be a helpful, and often more intuitive, way of coping with anxiety and other symptoms of mental illness.

Sleep

Lastly, one of the best ways that any of us can try to improve our mental health is to change our sleeping habits. Disrupted sleep can be a mental disorder in itself – one subset of the DSM-5 is dedicated to 'sleep–wake disorders', including insomnia and narcolepsy. But sleep disturbances weave their way through many other mental disorders, which makes sense given the wide-ranging impact sleep has on our psychological functioning. Sleep difficulties – such as trouble falling or staying asleep, sleeping too much, or sleeping a lot but still feeling tired – exacerbate just about every psychological process involved in mental illness. Poor sleep, particularly when chronic, affects the ability to regulate mood and to concentrate. Importantly, sleep problems not only accompany disorders like depression, anxiety and schizophrenia, they can *contribute* to their onset: longitudinal studies show that the sleep problems can come first, leading to an increased risk of subsequent mental disorder. Sleep disturbances therefore have a bidirectional relationship with symptoms of mental illness – poor sleep makes you more anxious, for example, but the state of being anxious makes it difficult to sleep, and the cycle continues.

Sometimes the solution to this is straightforward. Again, exercise can be helpful: people who exercise tend to sleep better, including those with mental illness. A review published in 2019 looked at eight studies in which people with various mental illness diagnoses, including depression, generalised anxiety disorder and PTSD, were randomly assigned to either an exercise intervention or a control group.[16] The exercise intervention varied between studies but included aerobic exercise, resistance training and yoga. Across studies, the authors found that the exercise condition had a large effect on subsequent sleep quality, and in some cases improved depressive symptoms too.

There are also so-called 'sleep hygiene' practices: a set of recommendations for healthy sleep, including advice on behaviour and the environment in which you sleep. It includes recommendations not to drink caffeine or alcohol close to bedtime, not to work in bed, and to ensure the bedroom is dark, for example. These tips are widely promoted in public health – they appear on the NHS website and are promoted in universities and schools. Interestingly, while there is evidence that individual components such as drinking less alcohol improve sleep in the general population, the evidence supporting sleep hygiene practices as a collective set of guidelines is somewhat mixed. Because there are many different components to sleep hygiene, some elements may be irrelevant to some people (e.g. those who don't drink anyway) or impossible to implement (those doing shift work), meaning it's hard to decipher what the 'active' component or components might be.[17] Sleep hygiene has also been trialled as a treatment for insomnia, but again evidence for its effectiveness is mixed.[18] But for those who are struggling with their mental health and not giving sleep the priority it needs, sleep hygiene might be a useful place to start.

For those with more chronic or complex sleep problems, there are other, more intensive interventions. Sleep clinics can investigate and diagnose difficulties like sleep apnoea and narcolepsy. There is a version of CBT specifically for treating insomnia, CBT-I, which has a clear evidence base. It's effective for people who 'only' have insomnia, but it's also helpful for people who have insomnia alongside another disorder: a review published in 2014 found that CBT-I improved insomnia in patients with depression, anxiety disorders, PTSD and substance use disorders – and sometimes reduced the symptoms of those disorders too.[19] For those who cannot see a therapist, there are many online programs and apps. For example, Sleepio, developed at the University of Oxford, guides the user through the principles of CBT-I on their phone.

In sum, wherever we fall on the spectrum of mental health to mental illness, there might be things we can try to help manage our well-being or our symptoms. Sometimes, some of us will need medical intervention – for those who are most seriously unwell, long-term or lifelong support from mental health professionals is necessary. But for the rest of us, for the rest of the time, these relatively simple methods for managing how we feel – whether that's reaching out to support one another, practising techniques for relaxation, taking exercise with others or adopting best practice for a good night's sleep – should continue to be part of the public discussion around mental health.

You can't always make things better

But it's vital to remember that there will be times when, no matter what we try, we cannot control or eliminate psychological suffering. I recently met a psychotherapist who worked in a university counselling service, and I asked her if there had been an increase in demand in services at her university in the decade or so that she'd worked there. She said she hadn't especially seen an increase in volume or severity of problems, but she had noticed that students were now coming to her with a different expectation of what therapy could achieve. They were now coming with the hope that she could get rid of their anxiety entirely (it was often anxiety that was the problem). 'I wish I could!' she said to me. A greater part of her job now than in the past was to tell students that she could help them get some relief and manage their anxiety, but the goal of therapy – and life – is not to eliminate these feelings altogether.

Grief is the price we pay for love, the saying goes; I would add that all forms of psychological distress are the price we pay for being alive. Suffering is part of being human. This is a truth many of us, myself included, struggle to accept. Like everyone else, when I'm in pain, I want it to go away. And yet some pain simply cannot be controlled, and we must find ways to live alongside or through it. This is not a message that exists in the public conversation right now, and that's a disservice to everyone. No matter how cautiously we try to live, we are all going to come up against unavoidable darkness in our lives. We all need to know that sometimes distress is normal and cannot be fixed. *Of course,* we must do what we can to look after ourselves while it's happening. But let's not add to our suffering by worrying that there is something wrong with us for feeling bad. As the psychiatrist Stanley Kutcher writes:

> The increased public perception that being well means only having positive feelings is taking over the social discourse on mental health. When the measure of health is simply feeling good, negative emotions become a marker of being unwell ... Mental health is not a static concept wearing a big smile. There are good days and bad days, good weeks and bad weeks.[20]

I sincerely hope this can be part of our new conversation about mental health. Just as some aspects of mental disorder must be endured, so too must other forms of psychological distress. These experiences can be ugly and exhausting, for the sufferer and those around them. We should all take steps to look after ourselves and each other, but we can't avoid the truth: sometimes, we must learn to live alongside the unhappiness we cannot control.

Some stress can be a good thing

To turn this on its head: within reason, some degree of distress might actually be a good thing. Of course we should take sensible precautions to avoid dangerous or traumatic situations, but we shouldn't design our lives (or our children's lives) to avoid stress altogether. In fact, the evidence suggests a certain level of stress is better than none at all.

In particular, stress which is time-limited and allows the opportunity for recovery might be protective in terms of coping with future hardships. This has been referred to as 'stress inoculation' or 'psychological immunisation'.[21] The coping skills described earlier in this book need to be developed somehow, and the idea of stress inoculation is that (mildly) stressful challenges teach us ways to cope. When future stressors arise, we are then more likely to believe they are manageable. One study found that, in a group of young adults experiencing stress at work, the ones who had already experienced work stress as teenagers seemed to cope better. For the stress novices, the new work challenges negatively affected their self-esteem and mood; for the stress-experienced, this didn't happen.[22]

Another study, published in 2010, asked nearly 2,400 adults to report their lifetime exposure to major negative events (such as physical assault, bereavement and divorce) and well-being.[23] They answered these questions at five different time points between 2001 and 2004. The researchers found a U-shaped relationship between life stress and subsequent well-being: compared to those who had experienced no negative life events and those who had experienced many, the participants who had experienced *some* life stress showed the lowest levels of distress (and highest levels of life satisfaction). In addition, these people were less negatively affected by recent life stress compared to the other two groups. More specifically, the researchers said that the pattern may be best described as J-shaped, because the 'no stressful events' and 'many stressful events' groups were not the same: experiencing many stressful life events was more harmful than experiencing none at all. But it seems that a little bit of stress may be a good thing. Here are the authors reflecting on their findings:

> Although sheltering from stressors may temporarily protect against distress, it ... provides no opportunity to develop toughness and mastery and is unlikely to persist indefinitely, so when stressors are eventually encountered, individuals are likely to be ill-equipped to cope with them. The development of toughness and mastery is analogous to the development of physical fitness from aerobic exercise: excessive exercise exerts a harmful toll on the body, but fitness does not improve with inactivity.

This has important implications for thinking about how best to raise children and teenagers to build up their resilience. Intuitively we may wish to protect them from any stress, but this isn't necessarily beneficial. As Jonathan Haidt and Greg Lukianoff argue in *The Coddling of the American Mind*, 'overparenting' does not help children in the long run. Of course, this doesn't mean intentionally causing young people stress, but we also shouldn't solve all their problems for them or panic if something challenging happens. Even the richest and most rewarding lives are peppered with heartbreak and hardships that must sometimes be managed and endured. I hope that this message – the benefits of working through manageable life stress – can also be added to the new conversation about mental health.

Passing time

This occasional need for endurance brings me to my final point in this book: the importance of time. When discussing his fiction-writing and own experience of mental illness, the writer Matt Haig said that time is 'the ultimate theme', and I couldn't agree more.[24] When I first experienced depression, I remember asking GPs and therapists one thing: have you seen people who feel like me get better? I asked because at that moment, I really couldn't fathom it. An intrinsic part of depression is the inability to see your way out of it, the belief that it will last forever; that's part of what makes it so miserable and scary, and why it leads some people to take their own lives. When I was first unwell, a family member who had experienced depression herself came to stay with me for a few days. I remember clinging on to how normal she seemed, with hope and disbelief: she'd got dressed properly, she was chatting, she was *laughing* – a very hard thing to get my head around. I looked at her and I found it deeply difficult to comprehend that she had once felt like I did. It was so important to see: that first time round, I needed external evidence, from other people, that it was possible to get better. This is where public discussions and stories of recovery can be so helpful: they provide evidence that it's possible to feel utter hopelessness and then come back from it, to even feel happy.

But over time, I became my own evidence. Having been through several episodes of depression and experienced at least some relief in between, I started to build up my own bank of evidence that I could feel very bad, be entirely convinced that it's permanent, and then come out of it. Now when I feel myself slipping again, I can hold on to this. Even though every fibre of my being is trying to tell me otherwise, I *know* the despair is temporary, because it was before. As Haig says, 'Time is the thing that is bigger than depression and anxiety, and can disprove their lies.'

Time teaches that recovery is not linear. One of the therapists I saw told me this, and it's always stuck with me. You don't get better in a steady and consistent fashion, she explained. In fact, she drew me a diagram, with time along the X axis and mood along the Y. She drew a wavy line across the graph, with peaks and troughs. At first the troughs are long and deep; the peaks infrequent and shallow. Then, slowly, the peaks become higher and they last longer. You will still have bad days, or bad weeks, she said. But the idea is that gradually the depths will be less deep and you'll come out of them sooner; the peaks will get higher and last longer.

I found this diagram so helpful. I have drawn it many times myself for other people, on a piece of paper or with my finger in the air. In other words: it's okay, and normal, if you have a setback, another trough. You will have times when you think you're getting better and then you'll fall again: you'll have a panic attack, or a binge, or whatever it may be. It doesn't mean it's all unravelling again. Sometimes the whole thing will catch you completely off guard, and you'll feel like you're playing snakes and ladders, suddenly slipping back down to square one. But this is just what getting better looks like. And the more people that know it – not just the person suffering but their friends and family too – the better.

For those of us who experience mental illness, time is an essential part of our toolkit. When managing symptoms, time is as important as the medication and therapy and self-help I've described so far. This is partly because we can look back and remind ourselves that we have improved before. You learn not to panic when you have a dip. But time can sometimes be a treatment in and of itself. I continue to be amazed by how situations and relationships and pain continually shift, simply because of the undulating waves of time.

A reasonable number of cases of depression actually resolve themselves, with no intervention. I haven't made a big point about it here because if you're concerned about your mental health, you should absolutely seek professional help. But it's worth saying just once. A meta-analysis from 2013 by researchers in Australia investigated how many people 'spontaneously' remit from depression – that is, how many people had depression and then improved, dropping below the threshold for a depressive disorder – even though they had no treatment.[25] To answer this question, they looked at people who were in control groups in treatment studies, and people who were in cohort studies, of the type I've discussed already in this book. In both cases, levels of depressive symptoms were monitored in these individuals, but they received no treatment. The researchers found that 23% of these adults experienced remission from depression within three months. This increased to 32% after six months, and 53% in a year.

What we learn from this is not that treatment is unnecessary. Many of these people might well have benefited from proper treatment. And just because someone drops below the threshold of official disorder doesn't mean their symptoms have resolved entirely. But this information should reassure us. Sometimes, either in parallel with treatment or not, the main thing you have to do is just *wait*. That's awful, I know it is. But time can change everything, and sometimes the best thing you can do is just find a way to hold on.

On the beach

As a society, we are standing at the edge of an ocean. True knowledge about our psychology and our suffering is as wide and deep as the sea, yet we spend most of our time in the shallows. Across these chapters, we've ventured into the water and gone diving, exploring the many hidden depths of mental health and illness. We've seen just what a messy topic this is, and the fundamental humanity that exists in so much of our distress. Now we are returning to the surface, retreating to the water's edge to reflect on what we have found.

I hope what you see is different now. To be honest, what I see is different too. I started this book with a good understanding about mental health and illness, but I have learnt so much more along the way. There are no easy answers, but that's the point: this topic defies any simple explanation. To recognise its complexity puts us in a far better position than pretending any of this is easy.

When I started this final image, with me standing on the beach, I didn't realise where I was. But as I write this now I see where I am: I'm in Turkey, in the beautiful harbour village of Kas, where for me this all started. And I'm walking now, away from the water. I'm walking on the cluttered pavement, past the shops selling scarves and jewellery, past restaurants with their outdoor tables and gingham tablecloths, and past the supermarket where we bought crisps and wine and big bottles of water. I'm walking past the doctor's office where I was injected with Valium, and then, as the buildings begin to fall away, I'm walking along the path towards our apartment, the path where I struggled to breathe.

I'm back at the apartment now, back in that hot September night. Like some Ghost of Summers Past, I can see my twenty-year-old self, my friends sat around me on the sofas, trying to help. And I wish I could speak to her, to that girl, to me. I wish I could say to her what I would say to any of you today, if you're suffering too: it's going to get better. It won't magically go away, and it's going to take a lot of hard work, but it's going to get better. Because it did.

Acknowledgements

Books are never the result of one person alone, and while mine is the only name on this one's front cover, many people contributed to this project.

It was an encouraging conversation with Pete Etchells in early 2019 that convinced me I should try to write this book. I will always be grateful for that phone call, because Pete advised me to get the best literary agent possible, and that led me to Will Francis at Janklow & Nesbit. Will helped shape my initial idea into something far stronger – apparently 'mental health is confusing' isn't enough of a pitch-line for a book proposal – and those early conversations really helped me refine what I was trying to say. I am immensely grateful for his expert guidance, then and ever since.

One Will then led to another, to Will Hammond at The Bodley Head, and I am lucky to have written this book with an exceptional editor by my side. From the main message and structure of the book down to discussions about specific sentences, Will's intellectual creativity and thoughtful input have been invaluable. The book is better because of him.

The seeds of this project were planted far earlier, though, and my thinking about mental health has been informed and enriched by many mentors and colleagues. Academia often gets a reputation for being cold and cutthroat, but I have been fortunate to work with many brilliant, lovely people. Number one among them is my former PhD supervisor Essi Viding. From the beginning, Essi allowed and encouraged my academic scepticism, and she has taught me a great deal about mental health, research and writing. It has also been a pleasure to work with and learn from Geoff Bird, Sarah-Jayne Blakemore, Alice Gregory, Pat Lockwood, Eamon McCrory, Dean McMillan and Craig Neumann. I am indebted to them for thinking differently, for questioning the stories we are told, and for showing that academia can be a fun, supportive place to be.

Thank you to Vaughan Bell and Matthew Broome for early chats about this book. Their acute awareness of the humanity involved in mental distress and 'illness' has deeply informed my thinking on this subject. Thank you to Mark Rice-Oxley and Dirk Richter, who gave their time to be interviewed and share their thoughts with me. I am also grateful to all the people who read and commented on drafts or sections of this book, whose input and edits were so helpful: Rachel Earl, Chris Francis, Elif Gökçen, Alice Gregory, Phil Kelly, Camilla Nord, Essi Viding and Portia Webb.

In need of his own paragraph here is Jack Andrews, who helped so much with reading over drafts and giving feedback. In the final frantic weeks, Jack also helped me check many of the stats and details from the referenced studies. But more importantly, he has been a good friend: encouraging and interested through the long and lonely process of writing a book. Thank you to him, and others, who regularly asked those sweet words every writer needs to hear: *How is the book going?* Not well, of course, but it's great to complain about it, thank you.

Outside of academia, thank you to my Mum, Dad and brother, for being enthusiastic about this book and for looking after me when I was at my worst. Thank you to Helen, who dropped everything and stayed with me at the darkest point. To Elli, Katie and Portia, who were with me in Turkey that summer and remain among my closest friends: thank you for doing what you could then, and for continuing to make life so much better today. More broadly, thank you to all my pals who care about me and make me laugh, and who remind me that this book and mental health research are but one part of my life. You make my world go round, and I'm so grateful for you all.

I also want to acknowledge the professionals who helped me cope with my own experience of depression and anxiety. In particular, I want to thank Neera, the fourth therapist I saw and the first that made me believe I might get better. Ten years on, I still remember the things she said to me, and I am indebted to her forever. Thank you also to those who have helped me manage the chronic pain that has long blighted my life and made writing this book, at times, so challenging. To Phil and Matt, in particular – in a very practical way, it would have been difficult to write this without their help.

Finally, I will end these acknowledgements where I began the book, with the boyfriend I mentioned in the opening paragraph. Mark, you were entirely unfazed, and so endlessly supportive, when your uni girl-friend of four months had a mental breakdown. You stayed by my side then, and through so many chapters and changes, you're still here now. Thank you for always listening, for making me laugh so much, and – most importantly – for staying the hell away while I wrote this book. It's all been possible because of you.

Notes

Introduction: Collateral damage

1   Woods, J. I have Obsessive–Christmas Disorder – and it's the greatest gift of all. *Telegraph* (2016).
2   Radomsky, A. S. et al. Part 1 – You can run but you can't hide: Intrusive thoughts on six continents. *Journal of Obsessive–Compulsive and Related Disorders* 3, 269–79 (2014).
3   Tuhus-Dubrow, R. 'Do I Really Want to Hurt My Baby?' Inside the disturbing thoughts that haunt new parents. *The Cut* (2018).
4   Torres, A. R. et al. Obsessive–Compulsive Disorder: Prevalence, Comorbidity, Impact, and Help-Seeking in the British National Psychiatric Morbidity Survey of 2000. *AJP* 163, 1978–85 (2006).
5   https://www.inquest.org.uk/natasha-abrahart-conclusion.
6   Aguirre Velasco, A., Cruz, I. S. S., Billings, J., Jimenez, M. & Rowe, S. What are the barriers, facilitators and interventions targeting help-seeking behaviours for common mental health problems in adolescents? A systematic review. *BMC Psychiatry* 20, 293 (2020).
7   Campbell, D. Mental health issues in young people up sixfold in England since 1995. *Guardian* (2018).
8   Friedman, R. A. Why Are Young Americans Killing Themselves? *New York Times* (2020).

Chapter 1: Rising rates

1   Iacobucci, G. NHS prescribed record number of antidepressants last year. *BMJ* 364, l1508. (2019).
2   OECD. Pharmaceutical consumption. *Health at a Glance 2017: OECD Indicators* (OECD Publishing, 2017).

3   Angold, A., Costello, E. J., Messer, S. C. & Pickles, A. Development of a short questionnaire for use in epidemiological studies of depression in children and adolescents. *International Journal of Methods in Psychiatric Research* 5, 237–49 (1995).

4   Thabrew, H., Stasiak, K., Bavin, L., Frampton, C. & Merry, S. Validation of the Mood and Feelings Questionnaire (MFQ) and Short Mood and Feelings Questionnaire (SMFQ) in New Zealand help-seeking adolescents. *International Journal of Methods in Psychiatric Research* 27, e1610 (2018).

5   Campbell, D. One in four girls have depression by the time they hit 14, study reveals. *Guardian* (2017).

6   Aftab, A. Conversations in Critical Psychiatry: Allen Frances, MD. *Psychiatric Times* vol. 36 (2019).

7   Busfield, J. Challenging claims that mental illness has been increasing and mental well-being declining. *Social Science & Medicine* 75, 581–8 (2012).

8   Richter, D., Wall, A., Bruen, A. & Whittington, R. Is the global prevalence rate of adult mental illness increasing? Systematic review and meta-analysis. *Acta Psychiatrica Scandinavica* 140, 393–407 (2019).

9   Schraer, R. Is young people's mental health getting worse? *BBC Reality Check* (2019).

10   Selby, E. A. et al. The dynamics of pain during nonsuicidal self-injury. *Clinical Psychological Science* 7, 302–20 (2019).

11   Van der Kolk, B. A. *The Body Keeps the Score: Brain, Mind, and Body in the Healing of Trauma* (Viking, 2014).

12   Hooley, J. M. & St. Germain, S. A. Nonsuicidal self-injury, pain, and self-criticism: Does changing self-worth change pain endurance in people who engage in self-injury? *Clinical Psychological Science* 2, 297–305 (2014).

13   MQ Open Mind podcast. Tackling the rise in self-harm among young people (2020).

14   Hooley, J. M. & Franklin, J. C. Why do people hurt themselves? A new conceptual model of nonsuicidal self-injury. *Clinical Psychological Science* 6, 428–51 (2018).

15   Patalay, P. & Gage, S. H. Changes in millennial adolescent mental health and health-related behaviours over 10 years: a population cohort comparison study. *International Journal of Epidemiology* 48, 1650–64 (2019).

16   McManus, S. et al. Prevalence of non-suicidal self-harm and service contact in England, 2000–14: repeated cross-sectional surveys of the general population. *Lancet Psychiatry* 6, 573–81 (2019).

17   Brampton, S. *Shoot the Damn Dog: A Memoir of Depression* (Bloomsbury, 2008).

18   World Health Organisation. *Suicide in the world: Global health estimates* (2019).

19   Arsenault-Lapierre, G., Kim, C. & Turecki, G. Psychiatric diagnoses in 3,275 suicides: A meta-analysis. *BMC Psychiatry* 4, 37 (2004).

20   Naghavi, M. Global, regional, and national burden of suicide mortality 1990 to 2016: systematic analysis for the Global Burden of Disease Study 2016. *BMJ* 364, l94 (2019).

21   https://www.who.int/news-room/fact-sheets/detail/suicide.

22   Office for National Statistics. *Suicides in the UK: 2018 registrations.* https://www.ons.gov.uk/peoplepopulationandcommunity/birthsdeathsandmarriages/deaths/bulletins/suicidesintheunitedkingdom/2018registrations (2019).

23 Hedegaard, H., Curtin, S. C. & Warner, M. *Suicide Mortality in the United States 1999–2017* (National Center for Health Statistics, 2018).

24 Pierce, M. et al. Mental health before and during the Covid-19 pandemic: a longitudinal probability sample survey of the UK population. *Lancet Psychiatry* 7, 883–92 (2020).

25 Richter, D. Personal communication (interview, 2020).

26 Wright, L., Steptoe, A. & Fancourt, D. Are we all in this together? Longitudinal assessment of cumulative adversities by socio-economic position in the first 3 weeks of lockdown in the UK. *Journal of Epidemiology and Community Health*, 74, 683–8 (2020).

27 Proto, E. & Quintana-Domeque, C. COVID-19 and mental health deterioration by ethnicity and gender in the UK. *PLOS ONE* 16, e0244419 (2021).

28 Kaseda, E. T. & Levine, A. J. Post-traumatic stress disorder: A differential diagnostic consideration for Covid-19 survivors. *The Clinical Neuropsychologist* 34, 1498–514 (2020).

29 Carmassi, C. et al. PTSD symptoms in healthcare workers facing the three coronavirus outbreaks: What can we expect after the Covid-19 pandemic. *Psychiatry Research* 292, 113312 (2020).

30 Dutheil, F., Mondillon, L. & Navel, V. PTSD as the second tsunami of the SARS-Cov-2 pandemic. *Psychological Medicine*, 1–2 (2020).

31 Lyons, D. et al. Fallout from the Covid-19 pandemic – should we prepare for a tsunami of post-viral depression? *Irish Journal of Psychological Medicine* 1–6 (2020).

32 Adam, D. The hellish side of handwashing: How coronavirus is affecting people with OCD. *Guardian* (2020).

33 Banerjee, D. The other side of Covid-19: Impact on obsessive–compulsive disorder (OCD) and hoarding. *Psychiatry Research* 288, 112966 (2020).

Chapter 2: On a continuum

1 Curtis, S. *It's Not OK to Feel Blue (and other lies)* (Penguin, 2019).

2 Beavan, V., Read, J. & Cartwright, C. The prevalence of voice-hearers in the general population: A literature review. *Journal of Mental Health* 20, 281–92 (2011).

3 Bell, V., Halligan, P. & Ellis, H. Beliefs about delusions. *The Psychologist* vol. 16, 418–22 (2003).

4 Freeman, D. et al. Psychological investigation of the structure of paranoia in a non-clinical population. *British Journal of Psychiatry* 186, 427–35 (2005).

5 Elahi, A., Perez Algorta, G., Varese, F., McIntyre, J. C. & Bentall, R. P. Do paranoid delusions exist on a continuum with subclinical paranoia? A multi-method taxometric study. *Schizophrenia Research* 190, 77–81 (2017).

6 *Diagnostic and Statistical Manual of Mental Disorders: DSM-5* (American Psychiatric Association, 2013).

7 Styron, W. *Darkness Visible: A Memoir of Madness* (Random House, 1990).

8 Rice-Oxley, M. *Underneath the Lemon Tree: A Memoir of Depression and Recovery* (Little, Brown, 2012).

9 Zimmerman, M., Ellison, W., Young, D., Chelminski, I. & Dalrymple, K. How many different ways do patients meet the diagnostic criteria for major depressive disorder? *Comprehensive Psychiatry* 56, 29–34 (2015).

10 Harald, B. & Gordon, P. Meta-review of depressive subtyping models. *Journal of Affective Disorders* 139, 126–40 (2012).

11 Wang, E. W. *The Collected Schizophrenias* (Graywolf Press, 2019).

Chapter 3: Moving goalposts

1   Surís, A., Holliday, R. & North, C. The evolution of the classification of psychiatric disorders. *Behavioral Sciences* 6, 5 (2016).

2   Van der Kloet, D. & van Heugten, T. The classification of psychiatric disorders according to DSM-5 deserves an internationally standardized psychological test battery on symptom level. *Frontiers in Psychology* 6, (2015).

3   Blashfield, R. K., Keeley, J. W., Flanagan, E. H. & Miles, S. R. The cycle of classification: DSM-I through DSM-5. *Annual Review of Clinical Psychology* 10, 25–51 (2014).

4   Haslam, N. Looping effects and the expanding concept of mental disorder. *Journal of Psychopathology* 22, 4–9 (2016).

5   Haslam, N. Concept creep: Psychology's expanding concepts of harm and pathology. *Psychological Inquiry* 27, 1–17 (2016).

6   Hjeltnes, A., Moltu, C., Schanche, E. & Binder, P.-E. What brings you here? Exploring why young adults seek help for social anxiety. *Qualitative Health Research* 26, 1705–20 (2016).

7   Mohammadi, A. et al. Cultural aspects of social anxiety disorder: A qualitative analysis of anxiety experiences and interpretation. *Iranian Journal of Psychiatry* 14, 33–9 (2019).

8   Gladwell, H. I spent thousands covering my body in tattoos during a bipolar mania episode – but I don't regret it. *Independent* (2019).

9   Misra, M., Greenberg, N., Hutchinson, C., Brain, A. & Glozier, N. Psychological impact upon London Ambulance Service of the 2005 bombings. *Occupational Medicine* 59, 428–33 (2009).

10 Bell, V. Let's not make a trauma out of a crisis. *Guardian* (2015).

11 Weathers, F. W. & Keane, T. M. The Criterion A problem revisited: Controversies and challenges in defining and measuring psychological trauma. *Journal of Traumatic Stress* 20, 107–21 (2007).

12 Hagan, M. J., Sladek, M. R., Luecken, L. J. & Doane, L. D. Event-related clinical distress in college students: Responses to the 2016 US Presidential election. *Journal of American College Health* 68, 21–5 (2020).

13 Roos, L. G., O'Connor, V., Canevello, A. & Bennett, J. M. Post-traumatic stress and psychological health following infidelity in unmarried young adults. *Stress and Health* 35, 468–79 (2019).

14 Gottlieb, L. Dear therapist: My girlfriend had an affair with my co-worker. *The Atlantic* (2019).

15 Sondel, B., Baggett, H. C. & Dunn, A. H. 'For millions of people, this is real trauma': A pedagogy of political trauma in the wake of the 2016 US Presidential election. *Teaching and Teacher Education* 70, 175–85 (2018).

16 Dowrick, C. & Frances, A. Medicalising unhappiness: new classification of depression risks more patients being put on drug treatment from which they will not benefit. *BMJ* 347, f7140 (2013).

17 Pies, R. W. The bereavement exclusion and DSM-5: An update and commentary. *Innovations in Clinical Neuroscience* 11, 19–22 (2014).

18 Fabiano, F. & Haslam, N. Diagnostic inflation in the DSM: A meta-analysis of changes in the stringency of psychiatric diagnosis from DSM-III to DSM-5. *Clinical Psychology Review* 80, 101889 (2020).

19 Aftab, A. Conversations in Critical Psychiatry: Allen Frances, MD. *Psychiatric Times* vol. 36 (2019).

20 Caspi, A. & Moffitt, T. E. All for one and one for all: Mental disorders in one dimension. *American Journal of Psychiatry* 175, 831–44 (2018).

21 Ibid.

22 Mansell, W., Harvey, A., Watkins, E. R. & Shafran, R. Cognitive behavioral processes across psychological disorders: A review of the utility and validity of the transdiagnostic approach. *International Journal of Cognitive Therapy* 1, 181–91 (2008).

23 Kendler, K. S. The nature of psychiatric disorders. *World Psychiatry* 15, 5–12 (2016).

24 Mattelaer, J. J. & Jilek, W. Sexual Medicine History: *Koro* – The Psychological Disappearance of the Penis. *The Journal of Sexual Medicine* 4, 1509–15 (2007).

25 Chowdhury, A. N. Dysmorphic penis image perception: The root of *Koro* vulnerability. *Acta Psychiatrica Scandinavica* 80, 518–20 (1989).

26 Ilechukwu, S. T. C. Magical penis loss in Nigeria: Report of a recent epidemic of a *Koro*-like syndrome. *Transcultural Psychiatric Research Review* 29, 91–108 (1992).

27 Kaiser, B. N. et al. *Reflechi twòp* – thinking too much: Description of a cultural syndrome in Haiti's Central Plateau. *Culture, Medicine, and Psychiatry* 38, 448–72 (2014).

28 Lee, J., Wachholtz, A. & Choi, K.-H. A review of the Korean cultural syndrome *Hwa-Byung*: Suggestions for theory and intervention. *Asia T'aep'yongyang Sangdam Yon'gu* 4, 49 (2014).

29 Kaiser, B. N. & Jo Weaver, L. Culture-bound syndromes, idioms of distress, and cultural concepts of distress: New directions for an old concept in psychological anthropology. *Transcultural Psychiatry* 56, 589–98 (2019).

Chapter 4: Biology

1 https://www.amacad.org/publication/unequal-nature-geneticists-perspective-human-differences.

2 Schizophrenia Working Group of the Psychiatric Genomics Consortium et al. Biological insights from 108 schizophrenia-associated genetic loci. *Nature* 511, 421–7 (2014).

3 Wray, N. R. et al. Genome-wide association analyses identify 44 risk variants and refine the genetic architecture of major depression. *Nature Genetics* 50, 668–81 (2018).

4 Howard, D. M. et al. Genome-wide meta-analysis of depression identifies 102 independent variants and highlights the importance of the prefrontal brain regions. *Nature Neuroscience* 22, 343–52 (2019).

5 Border, R. et al. No support for historical candidate gene or candidate gene-by-interaction hypotheses for major depression across multiple large samples. *American Journal of Psychiatry* 176, 376–87 (2019).

6 Watson, H. J. et al. Genome-wide association study identifies eight risk loci and implicates metabo-psychiatric origins for anorexia nervosa. *Nature Genetics* 51, 1207–14 (2019).

7   Smoller, J. W. et al. Psychiatric genetics and the structure of psychopathology. *Molecular Psychiatry* 24, 409–20 (2019).

8   Pingault, J.-B. et al. Genetic and Environmental Influences on the Developmental Course of Attention-Deficit/Hyperactivity Disorder Symptoms From Childhood to Adolescence. *JAMA Psychiatry* 72, 651–8 (2015); Pingault, J.-B., Rijsdijk, F., Zheng, Y., Plomin, R. & Viding, E. Developmentally dynamic genome: Evidence of genetic influences on increases and decreases in conduct problems from early childhood to adolescence. *Scientific Reports* 5, 10053 (2015).

9   Smoller, J. W. et al. Psychiatric genetics and the structure of psychopathology. *Molecular Psychiatry* 24, 409–20 (2019).

10   Insel, T. R. & Cuthbert, B. N. Brain disorders? Precisely. *Science* 348, 499–500 (2015).

11   Barch, D. M. Brain network interactions in health and disease. *Trends in Cognitive Sciences* 17, 603–5 (2013).

12   Menon, V. Large-scale brain networks and psychopathology: A unifying triple network model. *Trends in Cognitive Sciences* 15, 483–506 (2011).

13   Hamilton, J. P., Farmer, M., Fogelman, P. & Gotlib, I. H. Depressive rumination, the default mode network, and the dark matter of clinical neuroscience. *Biological Psychiatry* 78, 224–30 (2015).

14   Menon, V. & Uddin, L. Q. Saliency, switching, attention and control: A network model of insula function. *Brain Structure and Function* 214, 655–67 (2010).

15   Palaniyappan, L., White, T. P. & Liddle, P. F. The concept of salience network dysfunction in schizophrenia: From neuroimaging observations to therapeutic opportunities. *Current Topics in Medicinal Chemistry* 12, 2324–38 (2012).

16   Uddin, L. Q. & Menon, V. The anterior insula in autism: Under-connected and under-examined. *Neuroscience & Biobehavioral Reviews* 33, 1198–203 (2009).

17   Borsboom, D., Cramer, A. & Kalis, A. Brain disorders? Not really ... Why network structures block reductionism in psychopathology research. *Behavioral and Brain Sciences* 1–54 (2018).

18   Kaye, W. H., Wierenga, C. E., Bailer, U. F., Simmons, A. N. & Bischoff-Grethe, A. Nothing tastes as good as skinny feels: the neurobiology of anorexia nervosa. *Trends in Neurosciences* 36, 110–20 (2013).

19   Hay, P. J. & Sachdev, P. Brain dysfunction in anorexia nervosa: cause or consequence of under-nutrition? *Current Opinion in Psychiatry* 24, 251–6 (2011).

20   Toenders, Y. J. et al. Neuroimaging predictors of onset and course of depression in childhood and adolescence: A systematic review of longitudinal studies. *Developmental Cognitive Neuroscience* 39, 100700 (2019).

21   Steinglass, J. E. & Walsh, B. T. Neurobiological model of the persistence of anorexia nervosa. *Journal of Eating Disorders* 4, 19 (2016).

22   Barahona-Corrêa, J. B., Camacho, M., Castro-Rodrigues, P., Costa, R. & Oliveira-Maia, A. J. From thought to action: How the interplay between neuroscience and phenomenology changed our understanding of obsessive–compulsive disorder. *Frontiers in Psychology* 6, 1798 (2015).

23   Fried, E. I. & Kievit, R. A. The volumes of subcortical regions in depressed and healthy individuals are strikingly similar: a reinterpretation of the results by Schmaal et al. *Molecular Psychiatry* 21, 724–5 (2016).

24   Fried, E. All mental disorders are brain disorders ... not. https://eiko-fried.com/all-mental-disorders-are-brain-disorders-not (2020).

25   https://www.mqmentalhealth.org/articles/research-funding-landscape.

26   Kingdon, D. Why hasn't neuroscience delivered for psychiatry? *BJPsych Bulletin* 44, 107–9 (2020).

Chapter 5: Environment

1 Lieb, R. et al. Parental psychopathology, parenting styles, and the risk of social phobia in offspring: A prospective-longitudinal community study. *Archives of General Psychiatry* 57, 859–66 (2000).

2 Wang, E. W. *The Collected Schizophrenias* (Graywolf Press, 2019).

3 Children's Bureau. *Child Maltreatment 2007.* https://www.acf.hhs.gov/sites/default/files/cb/cm07.pdf (2007).

4 Stoltenborgh, M., Bakermans-Kranenburg, M. J., Alink, L. R. A. & van IJzendoorn, M. H. The prevalence of child maltreatment across the globe: Review of a series of meta-analyses. *Child Abuse Review* 24, 37–50 (2015).

5 Child Welfare Information Gateway. *Child abuse and neglect fatalities 2018: Statistics and interventions.* (2020).

6 Chen, L. P. et al. Sexual abuse and lifetime diagnosis of psychiatric disorders: Systematic review and meta-analysis. *Mayo Clinic Proceedings* 85, 618–29 (2010).

7 Norman, R. E. et al. The long-term health consequences of child physical abuse, emotional abuse, and neglect: A systematic review and meta-analysis. *PLoS Medicine* 9, e1001349 (2012).

8 McCrory, E. J. & Viding, E. The theory of latent vulnerability: Reconceptualizing the link between childhood maltreatment and psychiatric disorder. *Development and Psychopathology* 27, 493–505 (2015).

9 Manfro, G. Relationship of antecedent stressful life events to childhood and family history of anxiety and the course of panic disorder. *Journal of Affective Disorders* 41, 135–9 (1996).

10 Blazer, D., Hughes, D. & George, L. K. Stressful life events and the onset of a generalized anxiety syndrome. *American Journal of Psychiatry* 144, 1178–83 (1987).

11 Francis, J. L., Moitra, E., Dyck, I. & Keller, M. B. The impact of stressful life events on relapse of generalized anxiety disorder. *Depression and Anxiety* 29, 386–91 (2012).

12 Van der Kolk, B. A. *The Body Keeps the Score: Brain, Mind, and Body in the Healing of Trauma* (Viking, 2014).

13 McCrory, E. J. et al. Heightened neural reactivity to threat in child victims of family violence. *Current Biology* 21, R947–R948 (2011).

14 Kendler, K. S., Hettema, J. M., Butera, F., Gardner, C. O. & Prescott, C. A. Life event dimensions of loss, humiliation, entrapment, and danger in the prediction of onsets of major depression and generalized anxiety. *Archives of General Psychiatry* 60, 789–96 (2003).

15 Duncan, R. D. Maltreatment by parents and peers: The relationship between child abuse, bully victimization, and psychological distress. *Child Maltreatment* 4, 45–55 (1999).

16 Kuo, J. R., Khoury, J. E., Metcalfe, R., Fitzpatrick, S. & Goodwill, A. An examination of the relationship between childhood emotional abuse and borderline personality disorder features: The role of difficulties with emotion regulation. *Child Abuse & Neglect* 39, 147–55 (2015).

17 Bhugra, D. et al. Incidence and outcome of schizophrenia in Whites, African-Caribbeans and Asians in London. *Psychological Medicine* 27, 791–8 (1997).

18 Breslau, N. et al. Trauma and post-traumatic stress disorder in the community: The 1996 Detroit Area Survey of Trauma. *Archives of General Psychiatry* 55, 626–32 (1998).

19 Dick, D. M. Gene-environment interaction in psychological traits and disorders. *Annual Review of Clinical Psychology* 7, 383–409 (2011).

20 Farchione, T. J. et al. Unified protocol for transdiagnostic treatment of emotional disorders: A randomized controlled trial. *Behavior Therapy* 43, 666–78 (2012).

21 Olff, M., Langeland, W. & Gersons, B. P. R. The psychobiology of PTSD: coping with trauma. *Psychoneuroendocrinology* 30, 974–82 (2005).

22 Taylor, S. et al. Covid stress syndrome: Concept, structure, and correlates. *Depression and Anxiety* 37, 706–14 (2020).

23 Asmundson, G. J. G. et al. Do pre-existing anxiety-related and mood disorders differentially impact Covid-19 stress responses and coping? *Journal of Anxiety Disorders* 74, 102271 (2020).

24 Frankl, V. E. *Man's Search for Meaning: The Classic Tribute to Hope from the Holocaust* (Rider, 2004).

25 Laing, R. D. *The Divided Self: An Existential Study in Sanity and Madness* (Penguin Classics, 2010).

26 Laing, R. D. *The Politics of Experience and the Bird of Paradise* (Penguin Books, 1990).

27 'I knew I was in the right place': One on one ... with Lucy Johnstone. *The Psychologist* vol. 29, 732 (2016).

28 Hari, J. *Lost Connections: Uncovering the real causes of depression – and the unexpected solutions* (Bloomsbury, 2018).

29 Hari, J. Is everything you think you know about depression wrong? *Observer* (2018).

30 Borsboom, D. A network theory of mental disorders. *World Psychiatry* 16, 5–13 (2017).

31 Corcoran, C. et al. The stress cascade and schizophrenia: Etiology and onset. *Schizophrenia Bulletin* 29, 671–92 (2003).

Chapter 6: Adolescence

1   Kim-Cohen, J. et al. Prior juvenile diagnoses in adults with mental disorder: Developmental follow-back of a prospective-longitudinal cohort. *Archives of General Psychiatry* 60, 709–17 (2003).

2   Kessler, R. C. et al. Lifetime prevalence and age-of-onset distributions of DSM-IV disorders in the National Comorbidity Survey Replication. *Archives of General Psychiatry* 62, 593–602 (2005).

3   https://www.nhs.uk/conditions/early-or-delayed-puberty/.

4   https://www.who.int/maternal_child_adolescent/documents/second-decade/en/.

5   Blakemore, S.-J. Personal communication (email, 2020).

6   Schoen, R. & Baj, J. Twentieth-century cohort marriage and divorce in England and Wales. *Population Studies* 38, 439–49 (1984). Office for National Statistics. *Marriages in England and Wales: 2016.* https://www.ons.gov.uk/peoplepopulationandcommunity/birthsdeathsandmarriages/marriagecohabitationandcivilpartnerships/bulletins/marriagesinenglandandwalesprovisional/2016 (2019).

7   Sawyer, S. M., Azzopardi, P. S., Wickremarathne, D. & Patton, G. C. The age of adolescence. *Lancet Child & Adolescent Health* 2, 223–8 (2018).

8   Hayward, C. et al. Pubertal stage and panic attack history in sixth- and seventh-grade girls. *American Journal of Psychiatry* 149, 1239–43 (1992).

9   Tolentino, J. *Trick Mirror: Reflections on Self-delusion* (Random House, 2020).

10 Killen, J. D. Is puberty a risk factor for eating disorders? *Archives of Pediatrics & Adolescent Medicine* 146, 323–5 (1992).

11 Klump, K. L. Puberty as a critical risk period for eating disorders: A review of human and animal studies. *Hormones and Behavior* 64, 399–410 (2013).

12 Mendle, J., Turkheimer, E. & Emery, R. E. Detrimental psychological outcomes associated with early pubertal timing in adolescent girls. *Developmental Review* 27, 151–71 (2007).

13 Mendle, J. Why puberty matters for psychopathology. *Child Development Perspectives* 8, 218–22 (2014).

14 Nelson, E. E., Leibenluft, E., McClure, E. B. & Pine, D. S. The social reorientation of adolescence: A neuroscience perspective on the process and its relation to psychopathology. *Psychological Medicine* 35, 163–74 (2005).

15 Montemayor, R. & Eisen, M. The development of self-conceptions from childhood to adolescence. *Developmental Psychology* 13, 314–19 (1977).

16 Blakemore, S.-J. *Inventing Ourselves: The Secret Life of the Teenage Brain* (Doubleday, 2018).

17 Rapee, R. M. et al. Adolescent development and risk for the onset of social-emotional disorders: A review and conceptual model. *Behaviour Research and Therapy* 123, 1–14 (2019).

18 Sebastian, C., Viding, E., Williams, K. D. & Blakemore, S.-J. Social brain development and the affective consequences of ostracism in adolescence. *Brain and Cognition* 72, 134–45 (2010).

19 Zadro, L., Williams, K. D. & Richardson, R. How low can you go? Ostracism by a computer is sufficient to lower self-reported levels of belonging, control, self-esteem, and meaningful existence. *Journal of Experimental Social Psychology* 40, 560–7 (2004).

20 Sebastian, C. L. et al. Developmental influences on the neural bases of responses to social rejection: Implications of social neuroscience for education. *NeuroImage* 57, 686–94 (2011).

21 Burnett, S., Bird, G., Moll, J., Frith, C. & Blakemore, S.-J. Development during adolescence of the neural processing of social emotion. *Journal of Cognitive Neuroscience* 21, 1736–50 (2009).

22 Raihani, N. J. & Bell, V. An evolutionary perspective on paranoia. *Nature Human Behaviour* 3, 114–21 (2019).

23 Carskadon, M. A., Acebo, C. & Jenni, O. G. Regulation of adolescent sleep: Implications for behavior. *Annals of the New York Academy of Sciences* 1021, 276–91 (2004).

24 Wittmann, M., Dinich, J., Merrow, M. & Roenneberg, T. Social jetlag: Misalignment of biological and social time. *Chronobiology International* 23, 497–509 (2006).

25 Murnane, E. L., Abdullah, S., Matthews, M., Choudhury, T. & Gay, G. Social (media) jet lag: How usage of social technology can modulate and reflect circadian rhythms. *Proceedings of the 2015 ACM International Joint Conference on Pervasive and Ubiquitous Computing* 843–54 (ACM Press, 2015).

26 Baum, K. T. et al. Sleep restriction worsens mood and emotion regulation in adolescents. *Journal of Child Psychology and Psychiatry* 55, 180–90 (2014).

27 Paus, T., Keshavan, M. & Giedd, J. N. Why do many psychiatric disorders emerge during adolescence? *Nature Reviews Neuroscience* 9, 947–57 (2008).

Chapter 7: Social media

1 Barrie, J. Suicide rate almost doubles among teenagers, as social media giants are told they have a 'duty of care' to tackle it. *i* (2019).

2   Furness, H. Prince Harry says social media is more addictive than drugs as he condemns 'irresponsible' games. *Telegraph* (2019).

3   Twenge, J. M., Joiner, T. E., Rogers, M. L. & Martin, G. N. Increases in depressive symptoms, suicide-related outcomes, and suicide rates among US adolescents after 2010 and links to increased new media screen time. *Clinical Psychological Science* 6, 3–17 (2018).

4   Twenge, J. M. Have smartphones destroyed a generation? *The Atlantic* (2017).

5   Orben, A., Dienlin, T. & Przybylski, A. K. Social media's enduring effect on adolescent life satisfaction. *Proceedings of the National Academy of Sciences* 116, 10226–8 (2019).

6   Przybylski, A. K. & Orben, A. We're told that too much screen time hurts our kids. Where's the evidence? *Guardian* (2019).

7   Coyne, S. M., Rogers, A. A., Zurcher, J. D., Stockdale, L. & Booth, M. Does time spent using social media impact mental health?: An eight-year longitudinal study. *Computers in Human Behavior* 104, 106160 (2020).

8   Terán, L., Yan, K. & Aubrey, J. S. 'But first let me take a selfie': US adolescent girls' selfie activities, self-objectification, imaginary audience beliefs, and appearance concerns. *Journal of Children and Media* 14, 343–60 (2020).

9   Mills, J. S., Musto, S., Williams, L. & Tiggemann, M. 'Selfie' harm: Effects on mood and body image in young women. *Body Image* 27, 86–92 (2018).

10 Pool, E. How Has My Confidence Become Dependent On Instagram Likes? *HuffPost* (2019).

11 https://www.bbc.co.uk/news/av/uk-46966009.

12 Dodds, L. & Wright, M. Instagram removed nearly 10,000 suicide and self-harm images per day after the Molly Russell scandal. *Telegraph* (2019).

13 Jacob, N., Evans, R. & Scourfield, J. The influence of online images on self-harm: A qualitative study of young people aged 16–24. *Journal of Adolescence* 60, 140–7 (2017).

14 Luxton, D. D., June, J. D. & Fairall, J. M. Social media and suicide: A public health perspective. *American Journal of Public Health* 102, S195–S200 (2012).

15 Whitlock, J. L., Powers, J. L. & Eckenrode, J. The virtual cutting edge: The Internet and adolescent self-injury. *Developmental Psychology* 42, 407–17 (2006).

16 Lewis, S. P. & Seko, Y. A double-edged sword: A review of benefits and risks of online non-suicidal self-injury activities: Effect of online self-injury activities. *Journal of Clinical Psychology* 72, 249–62 (2016).

17 Branley, D. B. & Covey, J. Pro-ana versus pro-recovery: A content analytic comparison of social media users' communication about eating disorders on Twitter and Tumblr. *Frontiers in Psychology* 8, 1356 (2017).

18 Yau, J. C. & Reich, S. M. Are the qualities of adolescents' offline friendships present in digital interactions? *Adolescent Research Review* 3, 339–55 (2018).

19 Dolev-Cohen, M. & Barak, A. Adolescents' use of Instant Messaging as a means of emotional relief. *Computers in Human Behavior* 29, 58–63 (2013).

20 Davis, K. Friendship 2.0: Adolescents' experiences of belonging and self-disclosure online. *Journal of Adolescence* 35, 1527–36 (2012).

21 Wang, K. S., Smith, D. V. & Delgado, M. R. Using fMRI to study reward processing in humans: past, present, and future. *Journal of Neurophysiology* 115, 1664–78 (2016).

22 Van Geel, M., Vedder, P. & Tanilon, J. Relationship between peer victimization, cyberbullying, and suicide in children and adolescents: A meta-analysis. *JAMA Pediatrics* 168, 435–42 (2014).

23 Wolke, D., Lee, K. & Guy, A. Cyberbullying: A storm in a teacup? *European Child & Adolescent Psychiatry* 26, 899–908 (2017).

24 https://pessimists.co.

Chapter 8: Rethinking the crisis

1   Goodwin, M. Will Gen Z recover from Covid? *UnHerd* (2020).

2   Miller Beard, G. *American Nervousness, its Causes and Consequences: A Supplement to Nervous Exhaustion (Neurasthenia)* (Putnam, 1881).

3   McKay, B. & McKay, K. A Call for a New Strenuous Age. *The Art of Manliness*. https://www.artofmanliness.com/articles/call-new-strenuous-age/.

4   Moriarty, R. University bans litter pickers after snowflake students find them 'stressful'. *Sun* (2018).

5   Mahmood, B. Clapping banned at Oxford University to stop people being triggered. *Metro* (2019).

6   Du Toit, G. et al. Randomized trial of peanut consumption in infants at risk for peanut allergy. *New England Journal of Medicine* 372, 803–13 (2015).

7   Wingo, A. P., Baldessarini, R. J. & Windle, M. Coping styles: Longitudinal development from ages 17 to 33 and associations with psychiatric disorders. *Psychiatry Research* 225, 299–304 (2015).

8   Appleby, L. Personal communication (email, 2019).

9   McManus, S. et al. Prevalence of non-suicidal self-harm and service contact in England, 2000–14: repeated cross-sectional surveys of the general population. *Lancet Psychiatry* 6, 573–81 (2019).

10 Matthews, P. C. Epidemic of self-injury in an adolescent unit. *International Journal of Social Psychiatry* 14, 125–33 (1968).

11 Jarvi, S., Jackson, B., Swenson, L. & Crawford, H. The impact of social contagion on non-suicidal self-injury: A review of the literature. *Archives of Suicide Research* 17, 1–19 (2013).

12 Gould, M. S., Wallenstein, S., Kleinman, M. H., O'Carroll, P. & Mercy, J. Suicide clusters: an examination of age-specific effects. *American Journal of Public Health* 80, 211–12 (1990).

13 Hooley, J. M. & Franklin, J. C. Why do people hurt themselves? A new conceptual model of nonsuicidal self-injury. *Clinical Psychological Science* 6, 428–51 (2018).

14 Hamilton, I. Suicide rates match a spike in antidepressants. Look to austerity for the cause not lifestyle 'choices'. *Independent* (2019).

15 Office for National Statistics. *Suicides in the UK: 2018 registrations*. https://www.ons.gov.uk/peoplepopulationandcommunity/birthsdeathsandmarriages/deaths/bulletins/suicidesintheunitedkingdom/2018registrations (2019).

16 McCain, J. A. Antidepressants and suicide in adolescents and adults: A public health experiment with unintended consequences? *Pharmacy and Therapeutics* 34, 355–78 (2009).

17 Brent, D. A., Hur, K. & Gibbons, R. D. Association between parental medical claims for opioid prescriptions and risk of suicide attempt by their children. *JAMA Psychiatry* 76, 941–7 (2019).

18 Kutcher, S. Is my child depressed? Being moody isn't a mental illness. *The Conversation* (2018).

19 Hacking, I. Making Up People. *London Review of Books* vol. 28, no. 16 (2006).

20 Haslam, N. Looping effects and the expanding concept of mental disorder. *Journal of Psychopathology* 22, 4–9 (2016).
21 Summerfield, D. The invention of post-traumatic stress disorder and the social usefulness of a psychiatric category. *BMJ* 322, 95–8 (2001).
22 Furedi, F. The Cultural Underpinning of Concept Creep. *Psychological Inquiry* 27, 34–9 (2016).

Chapter 9: Language matters

1   Parkinson, H. J. 'It's nothing like a broken leg': Why I'm done with the mental health conversation. *Guardian* (2018).
2   Michelle Obama: Former US first lady says she has 'low-grade depression'. BBC News (2020).
3   Wheeler, K. What is low-grade depression? *Happiful* (2020).
4   Wisdom, J. P. & Green, C. A. 'Being in a funk': Teens' efforts to understand their depressive experiences. *Qualitative Health Research* 14, 1227–38 (2004).
5   Aguirre Velasco, A., Cruz, I. S. S., Billings, J., Jimenez, M. & Rowe, S. What are the barriers, facilitators and interventions targeting help-seeking behaviours for common mental health problems in adolescents? A systematic review. *BMC Psychiatry* 20, 293 (2020).
6   Summerfield, D. The invention of post-traumatic stress disorder and the social usefulness of a psychiatric category. *BMJ* 322, 95–8 (2001).
7   Smith, D. Alex Winter: 'I had extreme PTSD for many, many years. That will wreak havoc'. *Guardian* (2020).
8   http://www.lisamunro.net/blog-1/2017/5/14/leaving-academia-loss-grief-and-healing?utm_content=buffer477b6&utm_medium=social&utm_source=twitter.com&utm_campaign=buffer.
9   Curtis, S. *It's Not OK to Feel Blue (and other lies)* (Penguin, 2019).
10 Perkins, A. et al. Experiencing mental health diagnosis: a systematic review of service user, clinician, and carer perspectives across clinical settings. *Lancet Psychiatry* 5, 747–64 (2018).
11 https://www.kcl.ac.uk/events/58th-maudsley-debate-ptsd.
12 Office for National Statistics. *Suicides in the UK: 2018 registrations.* https://www.ons.gov.uk/peoplepopulationandcommunity/birthsdeathsandmarriages/deaths/bulletins/suicidesintheunitedkingdom/2018registrations (2019).
13 Stubley, P. Three in five secondary school pupils experience mental health problems, survey says. *Independent* (2019).
14 Rice-Oxley, M. Personal communication (interview, 2020).

Chapter 10: Expert help

1   Kan, K., Jörg, F., Buskens, E., Schoevers, R. A. & Alma, M. A. Patients' and clinicians' perspectives on relevant treatment outcomes in depression: Qualitative study. *BJPsych Open* 6, E44 (2020).
2   Pathak, A., Lim, E. & Lawrie, S. Needlessly controversial: The reporting of pharmaco- and psycho-therapy for the treatment of depression in the UK media. *Psychological Medicine* 1–6 (2020).
3   Kirsch, I. & Sapirstein, G. Listening to Prozac but hearing placebo: A meta-analysis of antidepressant medications. *Prevention & Treatment* 1, 303–20 (1998).

4   Kirsch, I. Antidepressants and the Placebo Effect. *Zeitschrift für Psychologie*, 222, 128–34 (2014).

5   Ibid.

6   Kirsch, I. *The Emperor's New Drugs: Exploding the Antidepressant Myth* (Bodley Head, 2009).

7   Cipriani, A. et al. Comparative efficacy and acceptability of 21 antidepressant drugs for the acute treatment of adults with major depressive disorder: A systematic review and network meta-analysis. *Lancet* 391, 1357–66 (2018).

8   Nord, C. Personal communication (email, 2020).

9   Cuijpers, P. et al. Adding psychotherapy to antidepressant medication in depression and anxiety disorders: a meta-analysis. *World Psychiatry* 13, 56–67 (2014).

10 Cuijpers, P. et al. A network meta-analysis of the effects of psychotherapies, pharmacotherapies and their combination in the treatment of adult depression. *World Psychiatry* 19, 92–107 (2020).

11 Barth, J. et al. Comparative efficacy of seven psychotherapeutic interventions for patients with depression: A network meta-analysis. *PLoS Medicine* 10, e1001454 (2013).

12 Gerger, H. et al. Integrating fragmented evidence by network meta-analysis: Relative effectiveness of psychological interventions for adults with post-traumatic stress disorder. *Psychological Medicine* 44, 3151–64 (2014).

13 Pompoli, A. et al. Psychological therapies for panic disorder with or without agoraphobia in adults: A network meta-analysis. *Cochrane Database of Systematic Reviews* (2016).

14 Skapinakis, P. et al. Pharmacological and psychotherapeutic interventions for management of obsessive–compulsive disorder in adults: A systematic review and network meta-analysis. *Lancet Psychiatry* 3, 730–9 (2016).

15 Cuijpers, P., Reijnders, M. & Huibers, M. J. H. The role of common factors in psychotherapy outcomes. *Annual Review of Clinical Psychology* 15, 207–31 (2019).

16 https://fivebooks.com/best-books/depression-bryony-gordon/.

17 Cuijpers, P., Reijnders, M. & Huibers, M. J. H. The role of common factors in psychotherapy outcomes. *Annual Review of Clinical Psychology* 15, 207–31 (2019).

18 NHS Digital. *Psychological Therapies: Reports on the use of IAPT services, England July 2020* (2020).

19 Campbell, D. Mental health care postcode lottery 'is risking lives'. *Observer* (2020).

20 Edbrooke-Childs, J. & Deighton, J. Problem severity and waiting times for young people accessing mental health services. *BJPsych Open* 6, e118 (2020).

21 Arie, S. Simon Wessely: 'Every time we have a mental health awareness week my spirits sink'. *BMJ* 358 (2017).

22 *Young, British and Depressed*. Channel 4, Dispatches (2019).

Chapter 11: Helping each other and ourselves

1   Bodie, G. D., Vickery, A. J., Cannava, K. & Jones, S. M. The role of 'active listening' in informal helping conversations: impact on perceptions of listener helpfulness, sensitivity, and supportiveness and discloser emotional improvement. *Western Journal of Communication* 79, 151–73 (2015).

2   Gould, M. S. et al. Evaluating iatrogenic risk of youth suicide screening programs: A randomized controlled trial. *JAMA* 293, 1635–43 (2005).

3   Polihronis, C., Cloutier, P., Kaur, J., Skinner, R. & Cappelli, M. What's the harm in asking? A systematic review and meta-analysis on the risks of asking about suicide-related behaviors and self-harm with quality appraisal. *Archives of Suicide Research* 1–23 (2020).

4   http://www.conversationsmatter.com.au/resources-community/someone-thinking-about-suicide.

5   https://www.samaritans.org/how-we-can-help/if-youre-worried-about-someone-else/supporting-someone-suicidal-thoughts/what-does-being-there-for-someone-involve/.

6   Nummenmaa, L., Glerean, E., Hari, R. & Hietanen, J. K. Bodily maps of emotions. *Proceedings of the National Academy of Sciences* 111, 646–51 (2014).

7   Van der Kolk, B. A. *The Body Keeps the Score: Brain, Mind, and Body in the Healing of Trauma* (Viking, 2014).

8   Rosenbaum, S., Tiedemann, A., Sherrington, C., Curtis, J. & Ward, P. B. Physical activity interventions for people with mental illness: A systematic review and meta-analysis. *Journal of Clinical Psychiatry* 75, 964–74 (2014).

9   Rees, D. I. & Sabia, J. J. Exercise and adolescent mental health: New evidence from longitudinal data. *Journal of Mental Health Policy and Economics* 13, 13–25 (2010).

10   ten Have, M., de Graaf, R. & Monshouwer, K. Physical exercise in adults and mental health status. *Journal of Psychosomatic Research* 71, 342–8 (2011).

11   Windle, F., Hughes, D., Linck, P., Russell, I. & Woods, B. Is exercise effective in promoting mental well-being in older age? A systematic review. *Aging & Mental Health* 14, 652–69.

12   Lubans, D. et al. Physical activity for cognitive and mental health in youth: A systematic review of mechanisms. *Pediatrics* 138, e20161642 (2016).

13   Manzoni, G. M., Pagnini, F., Castelnuovo, G. & Molinari, E. Relaxation training for anxiety: a ten-years systematic review with meta-analysis. *BMC Psychiatry* 8, 41 (2008).

14   Kremer, W. *The man who invented relaxation.* BBC World Service (2015).

15   Farias, M. & Wikholm, C. Has the science of mindfulness lost its mind? *BJPsych Bulletin* 40, 329–32 (2016).

16   Lederman, O. et al. Does exercise improve sleep quality in individuals with mental illness? A systematic review and meta-analysis. *Journal of Psychiatric Research* 109, 96–106 (2019).

17   Irish, L. A., Kline, C. E., Gunn, H. E., Buysse, D. J. & Hall, M. H. The role of sleep hygiene in promoting public health: A review of empirical evidence. *Sleep Medicine Reviews* 22, 23–36 (2015).

18   Chung, K.-F. et al. Sleep hygiene education as a treatment of insomnia: A systematic review and meta-analysis. *Family Practice* 35, 365–75 (2018).

19   Taylor, D. J. & Pruiksma, K. E. Cognitive and behavioural therapy for insomnia (CBT-I) in psychiatric populations: A systematic review. *International Review of Psychiatry* 26, 205–13 (2014).

20   Kutcher, S. Is my child depressed? Being moody isn't a mental illness. *The Conversation* (2018).

21   Seery, M. D., Holman, E. A. & Silver, R. C. Whatever does not kill us: Cumulative lifetime adversity, vulnerability, and resilience. *Journal of Personality and Social Psychology* 99, 1025–41 (2010).

22 Mortimer, J. T. & Staff, J. Early work as a source of developmental discontinuity during the transition to adulthood. *Development and Psychopathology* 16, 1047–70 (2004).

23 Seery et al., op. cit.

24 Sutton, J. 'It's about editing our lives so that they make sense again'. *The Psychologist* vol. 31, 48–9 (2018).

25 Whiteford, H. A. et al. Estimating remission from untreated major depression: a systematic review and meta-analysis. *Psychological Medicine* 43, 1569–85 (2013).

Index